The Medical Performance Management Manual:

How to evaluate employees

Second Edition

By:
Courtney Price, PhD
and
Alys Novak, MBA

Published by:
Medical Group Management Association
104 Inverness Terrace East
Englewood, CO 80112
Toll-free 877.ASK.MGMA
www.mgma.com

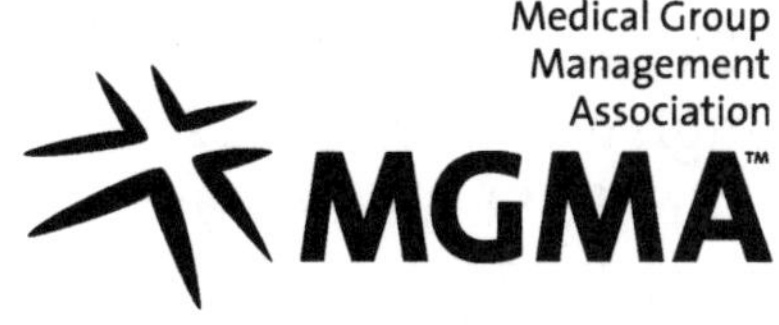

Medical Group Management Association
104 Inverness Terrace East
Englewood, CO 80112
ISBN #1-56829-146-9
Item #5786

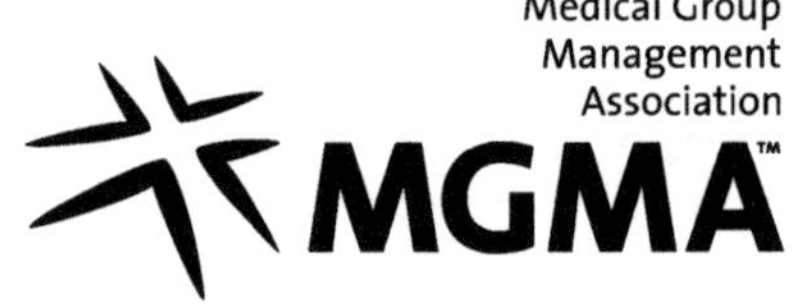

Table of Contents

Table of Contents

Table of Contents

Preface

The Medical Practice Performance Manual, first edition, remains a classic that you should continue to use as a key reference manual in developing and revising your performance management system. It contains proven management techniques and samples of exemplary performance evaluation tools, forms, developmental plans, performance interview checklists, self-appraisal worksheets, surveys and tips on supervisory training. It is the perfect companion to the second edition that includes the newest performance management thinking with the focus on managing and motivating the new workforce using self-management and coaching principles. This second edition contains numerous references to top Web sites that offer valuable performance management materials. (All Web references highlighted in the second edition were accurate at the time of printing.) Following the suggested guidelines in both manuals will enable you to build an effective performance management system for your group practice.

"Performance appraisal," "performance review," and "performance evaluation" are well known phrases and concepts for medical practice administrators and for managers in any field. The step of examining how employees are performing is a natural act for any supervisor, whether or not the step is formalized.

Unfortunately, when formalized, this step is often taken with an attitude of "have to" on the part of the supervisor. In turn, employees respond with a "do we have to?" feeling. Too often such reviews are yearly rituals with little thought or preparation – and little long-term meaning to either party. More important, they rarely change behavior for the better.

Fortunately, employee performance evaluation does not have to fall into this sinkhole. By switching gears to *performance management*, administrators can put the focus on steps that facilitate future success. They can put the emphasis on identifying performance expectations upfront, reinforcing them consistently and rewarding results regularly – and on making positive changes.

As spelled out in this text, current management philosophies place great weight on the upfront need to develop and improve the knowledge, skills, abilities and competencies of employees at all levels in an organization on an ongoing basis. The key strategy: constant communication throughout the work year about performance goals and results, rather than a once-a-year, after-the-fact event.

As medical practice managers tackle the challenges of the new century, they will find that integrating contemporary performance management tools and technology with classic techniques will make the difference when dealing with their most important asset – people. *The Medical Practice Performance Manual,* second edition, puts the spotlight on the power of self-management, coaching, mentoring, flexible work options, variable pay and other up-to-date methods for achieving performance goals in the 2000s.

About the authors

Courtney Price, PhD, is very familiar with the human resource management needs of medical group practices and industry trends. She wrote MGMA's first personnel policy manual in 1984 (*The Management Guide for Developing Personnel Policies, Procedures and Employee Handbooks*) which has been updated numerous times with the latest 1997 edition – *The Group Practice Personnel Policies Manual Management Guide for Developing Policies Manual* with policy examples on disk. She also authored the *Group Practice Job Description Handbook* series and co-authored with Alys Novak *the Medical Practice Performance Management Manuals* and *Tracking Hot HR Trends.* She also co-authored (with Bruce Stickler) *MGMA HR Issues* (formerly *Personnel Postscript*), a quarterly newsletter for human resource professionals. Price also has written numerous other management books focusing on implementing innovative ideas by igniting the entrepreneurial spirit within organizations. She is the president of VentureQuest, a consulting and training company that helps organizations create bottom-line profits and new revenue streams by capitalizing on developing people, technologies and market opportunities.

Alys Novak, MBA, is president of Discovery Communications, Inc., a communications and consulting/training firm. Her many assignments in the health care field have focused on medical practices, home health and rural health. Her fields of expertise include strategic planning, marketing, performance management and compensation. For many years she served as adjunct faculty at Metropolitan State College and the University of Colorado teaching a variety of business topics. She has co-authored several books including *User-Friendly Psychology for Medical Practices* and *Nonprofit Financial Management* and is the author of *Governing Policies for Medical Practices.* She co-authored *The Medical Practice Performance Management Manual* and *Job Description Manual for Medical Practices* with Courtney Price. Associated with MGMA for more than 20 years, she presently serves as its Acquisitions Editor. In addition, she is a project manager for the Visiting Nurse Corporation of Colorado.

Acknowledgments

The authors gratefully appreciate the help of the MGMA Information Center staff, especially Kristen Russell for her guidance and support.

Acknowledgment also goes to Mary Huey and Brian Novak who provided production assistance and to Orbit Design for the cover design.

In particular, the authors want to offer a special thank you to Cathleen Hight and Tara Powers. These fellow consultants contributed directly to the design, focus and content of the text. Their involvement and sharing of their expertise strengthened this book.

Overview

"One of the things company executives always ask is, 'How do we get employees to be more committed to the goals of the company and involved in the success of the company?' However, from the employee's viewpoint, the question is not 'How committed are we to the organization?' but, 'How committed is the organization to us?'"—Dr. Robert Eisenberger [1]

For performance management to be successful, organizations in this century will need to create strategic partnerships with their employees. All the efforts toward managing change, creating employee involvement, building teams and delivering top-notch patient care will not occur without managing individual performance levels of employees.

The fundamental processes and techniques of performance management work in all organizations and medical group practices. All employees want to know what's expected, how they are performing, and how they will be evaluated and recognized for their accomplishments. An effective performance management system provides a consistent process that keeps the practice focused on its goals and results and supports the growth and development of its most important investment and asset—its people.

What is Performance Management?

A formal definition may read, "Performance management is a scientific and data-oriented system that consists of measurement, feedback and positive reinforcement." In an everyday nutshell, ***Performance management is getting people to do what's best for the organization and to enjoy doing it.***

Imagine what it would be like if everyone in your group practice performed the best they could and enjoyed working together to accomplish the organization's goals? If performance management were working for your practice, you'd experience these end results:

- The staff would work as a team to manage the practice's operations and to provide excellent patient care;
- Staff members would understand their roles and the impact of their performance;
- Each staff member would be positively motivated to do his or her best;
- Patients would receive quality care and documentation would be timely;
- Billing information would be accurate and claims processed quickly; and
- The organization would consistently reach its goals.

Still a Standard

Classic reference serves as standard.

Follow-Up to the First Edition

The release of MGMA's *The Medical Practice Performance Management Manual: How to Evaluate Employees* in 1993 provided an excellent reference tool for managers and supervisors to review how performance was measured and managed in their practices. Since the release of this publication, many new ideas and strategies have been developed and incorporated in this updated edition.

While reflecting on many previous best practices, this second edition attempts to bring to health care organizations additional resources and techniques to enhance their performance management systems. For medical group practices that have yet to create and implement such a system, this book provides an up-to-date overview including winning strategies that have been used successfully by other group practices.

Quick Look

Chapter One explores many of the recent changes in the workplace. For starters, the workforce has become more diverse than ever and practices are learning how to manage employees who span a continuum of age, culture, values and lifestyles. Besides dealing with diversity, many organizations are also exploring new work options such as flextime, telecommuting and job sharing. Recognizing what's changed in the world of work helps to place performance management in a new perspective.

Chapter Two reviews best practices of attracting, retaining and developing talent in health care organizations. These are ongoing challenges for most organizations and for the health care industry in particular. Organization performance is primarily accomplished through people and while it is ideal to attract and retain the best talent, practices also have to focus on attracting "good" people and developing them into "stars."

Chapter Three provides an overview of a performance management process and a performance management system and the difference between the two. As a practice, you'll explore how employee performance is aligned with your organizational goals and how each component supports your performance management process.

Chapter Four explores the newest trends in performance management including: how important it is to support employees in managing their careers; how managers can coach for performance; and how mentoring can assist employees in meeting their performance goals.

Chapter Five reviews best practices related to implementing a successful performance management system that embraces effective goal setting, performance measures, ongoing feedback and regular evaluation of employee performance.

Chapter Six allows your practice to explore how to align compensation strategies with performance outcomes. The components of a total pay system are reviewed with an emphasis on performance-based pay plans. Implementing pay-for-performance strategies communicates a strong message that the practice rewards performance.

Chapter Seven explores the roles that recognition and rewards play in a performance management process. Guidelines for giving recognition and rewards for both individual and group performance are explained. Additional tips are provided about creating an incentive program for your practice.

Chapter Eight offers ongoing integration strategies for your practice's performance management process. Factors to consider include documentation and operating within legal guidelines to evaluate and reward employee performance. The use of online performance management systems and incorporating new hire orientation are also reviewed. Once your practice has implemented its system, ongoing evaluation of its effectiveness is important and is discussed.

Chapter Nine provides additional tips for managers and supervisors about their roles in ensuring a successful performance management system. Guidelines on maintaining leadership, gaining commitment, communicating outcomes and managing expectations are integral strategies your practice must include for ongoing success.

The concept of performance management is not new and many practices are learning and sharing how successful models take place. Hopefully, your practice is becoming its own "star" in the health care industry.

References

1. Dr. Robert Eisenberger, excerpted from his presentation at the Aubrey Daniels International Senior Executive Leadership Forum, pmezine.com (the performance management magazine online).

Changes at Work in the New Century

Chapter 1

In this chapter, we'll explore what's new in the workplace of the new century. First, we'll look at an increasingly diverse workforce that has materialized over the past couple of decades. Diversity is not just about race and gender. It includes a wide spectrum of differences, including age and education. A clash between multiple work generations is currently at hand as we see people working together whose ages range from 18 to over 80. Insights into managing four distinct generational groups will be shared.

Next, we'll review cultural diversity challenges and best practices for implementing diversity awareness. Cultural diversity is on the rise for three important reasons: (1) patient demographics are reflecting the changes relating to a global workforce; (2) health care organizations continue to face a shortage of "traditional" workers; and (3) organizations are striving to attract a workforce that understands its customers' cultural differences.

Then, this chapter explores alternative work options that organizations are using to manage the challenges and needs of the new workforce. As the health care industry continues to change to meet increasing demands and workforce challenges, managers and supervisors will be on the lookout for new ideas and solutions. The solutions start with understanding the new workforce and the workplace. It's definitely changed radically over time.

And finally, we'll take a brief glance at how performance management has changed to address a different workplace and a new workforce. A more in-depth study of performance process and system will be offered in the chapters that follow.

Four Generations at Work

- The Matures (born between 1922- 1943)
- Baby Boomers (born between 1943 - 1960)
- Generation X (born between 1961 - 1980)
- Generation Y or Millenials (74 million born after 1980)

The Increasingly Diverse Workforce

Today's workforce is more diverse than ever with a variety of races, genders, ethic groups and generations. These employees have different values, ambitions, perspectives and mindsets. An understanding of the issues that arise due to differences between age, religions, gender, sexual orientation, physical capabilities and cultures is needed to work harmoniously and bring out the best in all employees.

Multi-Generations

Although each element of diversity poses its unique challenges, generational diversity is difficult to manage in many organizations. Perhaps this is because for the first time in our work history, we have four unique generations working side by side throughout our organizations. In this new century, your staff and managers are learning to work with a more age-diverse crowd than ever before.

Each of these four generations has its own unique perspective about work, career, management and the organization as a whole. Understanding these generational differences is important to blend these different viewpoints with the values and objectives of today's health care organizations. By understanding more about each of the generational work groups, managers can learn how to transform generational differences into a competitive advantage for their organizations.

The four main generations that make up the work force span nearly 80 birth years from 1922 – 2000+. Although called by various titles, most diversity sources have named these four generations as the Matures, Baby Boomers, Generation X and Generation Y. They are differentiated by these demographics:

- Matures or Veterans (35 million people born between • 1922- 1943)
- Baby Boomers (76 million people born between 1943 - 1960)
- Generation X (60 million people born between 1961 - 1980)
- Generation Y or Millenials (74 million born after 1980)

The following descriptions provide an overview of each of the four distinct generational work groups and their different characteristics. Keep in mind that although these generalizations appear to be stereotypes, the reality is that there are exceptions to every categorization and these generalizations don't always hold true.

Matures, Veterans or Traditionalists (born between 1922 and 1943)

Matures account for about 25 percent of the workforce and their numbers are shrinking as they move into retirement. These elders are "keepers of the grail" and view themselves as important contributors to the practice. Matures view their employer as the Benevolent Master and are loyal and hard working. They are known as "company people" and tend to be more loyal and stay with their organizations the longest—often 15 to 25 years or more.

The misconception about Matures is that they: are set in their ways; are counting the days until retirement; don't deal well with ambiguity or change; and are uncomfortable with conflict. The truth is that most Matures enjoy trying new things if they have the time to learn. They can be good role models for younger generations and they have a deep respect for their employers and authority.

Baby Boomers (born between 1943 and 1960)

There are currently about 76 million Baby Boomers in North America alone. Although still a very active part of the workforce, they are slowly becoming the next group of employees to retire. Boomers grew up in an optimistic and positive era of the economy. They still believe in growth and expansion and think of themselves as the "stars of the show." Boomers are team players and open to all types of diversity.

At work, they want to be managers or work for managers who treat them as equals. Boomers want flexible work hours and work styles and have a strong need to be great parents and great employees. Remember, these were the workers who were at the forefront of revolutionizing the workforce, pushing for a more casual work environment and the ability to work from home.

The misconception about Baby Boomers is that they think primarily of themselves and their own personal needs. They have been dubbed the "Me" generation. Actually, Boomers are concerned about spirit in the workplace, bringing heart and humanity to the office, and creating a fair and level playing field for all.

Generation X (born between 1961 and 1980)

There are an estimated 60 million people in this generation. They grew up in the era of Watergate and the energy crisis. Half of them have divorced parents and were consequently a major wave of latchkey kids. Generation Xers, as they are sometimes called, have learned to be self-reliant and not to rely on close supervision. They sometimes have a nontraditional approach to work and tend to be casual about deadlines. Gen Xers are careful about loyalty and commitment because they've watched their parents suffer through the first waves of downsizing.

The great myth about Gen Xers is that they are "children," who jump from one job to the next and are only concerned about material wealth. The reality is that many Gen Xers have established careers with families of their own and work hard to find balance between work and home.

Generation Y, Echo Boomers, Nexters or Millenials (born post-1980)

This generation of approximately 74 million people is the newest to enter the work force. Gen Yers are the confident offspring of the most age-diverse group of parents—Xers and Boomers. There are almost as many Gen Yers as Boomers. Although there aren't many Gen Yers in your practice now, they will be one of the largest groups of employees in the next few decades.

The Generation Yers will resemble the Matures in many ways: they have a very strong work ethic; they believe in collective action; and they trust centralized authority. Both Gen Xers and Gen Yers have strong technical strengths. Gen Yers were born and raised in the Information Age and will bring the most technological change to the workplace.[1]

Managing Multiple Generations at Work

Although some practices are full of generational strife, many of them have learned how to harness the power and potential of their differences. Most of the misunderstandings between employees of different generations involve learning how to understand their differences and how to communicate with one another. By recognizing each generation's core values and motivators, as well as what they all have in common, managers can create a stronger workplace that leverages generational differences.

Randstad, an international employment solutions firm, conducted "The 2001 Employee Review" that revealed work expectations for each generational work group. Although there are key differences among the various generational work groups, Randstad noted that all four groups share these same work expectations:

- Being able to balance work and personal life;
- Having opportunities to try new things at work; and
- Doing their jobs successfully.

All Four Generations Have These Same Expectations:

1. Balancing work and personal life
2. Trying new things at work
3. Succeeding at their jobs

Overall, the Randstad study found that nine out ten employees wanted the same things—to achieve work satisfaction. This was defined as work that gives them personal satisfaction, work that is valued by their employer and customers, and work with an employer who understands that personal lives are important, too. Although money is a higher motivator for Gen Xers and Yers, they describe job satisfaction as being met by things other than money.[2] For many managers it's the differences among the four generational work groups that make it difficult to motivate employees. Each generational work group has specific core values and motivators that are important for managers and supervisors to know. Understanding the needs of each group and how to motivate employees to achieve peak performance will further enhance your practice's ability to reach its performance goals.

The table in Figure 1-1 provides an overview of each generational work group, their core values and what motivates them to perform. This represents a compilation of various sources who have reported on generational work differences.

Figure 1-1
Core Values and Motivators by Generation

Generation	Core Values	Motivators
Matures	• Respect and loyalty of peers. • Work on and work as part of a team. • The history and reputation of "their" company. • Stable and secure environment. • Develop a strong loyalty to the company. • Commitment, discipline, financial and social conservatism.	• Helping customers. • Mentoring others. • Sharing knowledge with co-workers and customers. • Knowing they make a difference. • Respect and trust from management. • The personal touch—handwritten notes, non-technical communication. • Flexible work schedules and personal time off. • Traditional perks—upfront parking spaces, plaques.
Baby Boomers	• Stable and secure future. • Benefit society and workplace. • Fairness and equity for all. • Social status. • Freedom from pressures to conform both on and off the job.	• Share company information and goals. • Balance between work and home. • Teamwork. • Involved in decision-making. • Public recognition of achievements. • The personal approach to being asked to do things. • More personal time off. • Career planning. • Financial benefits. • Perks—travel, car allowances, gifts.

Generation Xers	• Learn new things. • Teamwork and a sense of belongingness. • Ability to exercise leadership and a chance to use their abilities. • Contribute to important decisions. • Opportunities for advancement. • A variety of work assignments. • Stimulating and challenging work. • Immediate gratification—don't want to wait for things. • Have fun in their lives and at work.	• Training opportunities. • Allowances for personal time. • Flexible work schedules and ability to work from home. • Recognition for meeting goals. • More responsibility and career advancement opportunities. • Projects where they can use their skills. • Control over their own work. • Career planning.
Generation Yers	• Make a good living. • Interesting work challenges. • Teamwork. • Have fun in their lives and at work. • Learn new things. • Stability. • Traditions.	• Opportunities to work with co-workers in and out of the office. • Knowing the "big picture." • Teamwork. • Career development plan. • Training and a chance to learn new skills. • Individual bonuses and incentives for exceeding goals. • Ability to try new things on their own. • Flexible schedules and ability to work from home. • Less overtime and more personal time.

Helping Generations Work Well Together

Because your practice is looking for ways to help employees learn to work together more effectively, these approaches should help to make your work environment more comfortable and more motivating for all generations:

- Identify the main generational work groups in your practice and determine the needs of each group by asking:
  - *"What do you value the most in your workplace"*
  - *"What motivates you to perform?"*
- Provide ways for employees to talk openly about generational differences, their values and views about work—what they find most rewarding, their preferences for communication, and their strengths.
  - Offer a fun workshop about generational differences where employees create "generation groups" and compare one group to another in a non-threatening way.
  - Hold discussions where employees can talk about their work and personal values and their expectations of managers and co-workers.
  - Use these group discussions to help employees recognize their similarities. Employees usually discover they have more in common than originally anticipated.
- Learn what different employees value in their current work life by talking about their personal work needs and career plans. Then, provide benefits to meet different developmental needs (e.g., offer training to Generation Xers and Yers to develop new skills for advancement, allow Matures to work flexible hours to care for grandchildren).
- Use cafeteria-type incentive plans to better meet needs of the different generational work groups.
- Offer more flexibility in work schedules to allow employees to balance their work and personal lives.
- Offer training and development opportunities to further work and communication skills, including:
  - Learning to work with different behavior styles
  - Conflict resolution
  - Team building
- Leverage the strengths and needs of each generational work group by:

- Providing mentoring opportunities for Matures and other generational work groups.
- Having Matures share knowledge about the practice and the industry by having them manage new hire orientation.
- Letting Gen Xers and Yers share their technical knowledge and skills by having them coach other employees on how to use software applications.
- Creating project and team building opportunities for each generational work group to work together such as upgrading software on computers or planning a holiday party.

Three Ways to Create a Diverse-Friendly Work Atmosphere

1. Provide diversity training.
2. Humanize encounters.
3. Celebrate diversity.

Multi-Cultures

Over the past few decades, organizations have seen dramatic changes in the fabric of the workplace. Currently, 53 percent of the workforce is comprised of people of color, women and immigrants.[3] According to the Bureau of Labor Statistics, the number of Asian-Americans and Hispanics in the workforce will grow by 40 percent and 37 percent between 1998 and 2008. The black workforce is expected to grow 20 percent, which is twice as fast as the 10 percent growth rate for whites.[4]

As the dramatic shift to a highly diverse workforce continues, organizations know they must do a better job of helping all employees to understand, accept and capitalize on their differences. More and more practices are realizing that managing diversity in the workplace is good business and good for business.

Employee Demographics Mirror Those of Patients

The demographics of patients have changed along with the global workforce landscape. If health care organizations are to maintain high standards of patient care, they must be prepared to meet the challenges that our nation's increasingly diversity poses. Health care workers who understand other cultures can help to ensure medical compliance and are better able to communicate with minority patients. This type of sensitivity helps patients of all cultures to strive for optimal care and feel comfortable accessing health care benefits.[5]

Diversifying the health care workforce will help to increase the recognition and tolerance for diversity. Managing diversity starts with your organization's policy of hiring underrepresented minorities whenever possible. This is the first step toward embracing a diverse workplace.

Helping Your Practice to Manage Diversity

Here are three ways your practice can create a more diverse-friendly work atmosphere:

- Provide diversity training—Send a strong message that the practice values a diverse work culture. Addressing stereotypes individually, managerially and organizationally should be a part of the diversity change process because it's embedded in human behavior. If your practice doesn't have diversity training available, contact cultural organizations in your area, such as the Asian Center or the Hispanic Chamber of Commerce.
- Humanize encounters—Most stereotypes are generalizations based on limited experiences with individuals from different groups. If possible, mix employees across boundaries by creating ways for them to interact with one another. Assigning mixed groups to each project, cross-training and social/recreation activities can help employees to develop relationships across lines of difference.[6]
- Celebrate diversity—Find opportunities to recognize and learn about employees' cultures, religions and homelands. Have employees bring in pictures of where they're from, share stories about their families, or plan potluck lunches with each person bringing a favorite dish from their culture. Everyone is diverse in some way and the more employees learn about one another, the more likely they are to accept their differences.

Best Practices in Diversity

Many health care organizations have employed successful diversity initiatives to help their employees embrace their differences including:

- Holy Cross Hospital conducts a diversity gala each year and asks employees to place a pin on maps on the state or country where they were born. Displayed in a public place in the hospital, the United States and world maps reflect that employees are not only from 50 states but also from many countries.[7]

- Harvard Pilgrim Hospital offers a three-day diversity training that covers the gamut of diversity activities, including staged role-playing and community visits.
- Cross-Cultural Health Care Program, an independent Seattle-based group, conducts patient-centered ethnicity workshops.
- Kaiser Permanente integrates cultural sensitivity into a variety of continuing medical education courses on communicating with patients. [8]
- Blue Cross and Blue Shield of Minnesota actively recruits and retains minority employees by sponsoring job fairs targeted to diverse populations and linking with professional organizations that represent people of color.[9]

Practices that help their employees to tolerate diversity will benefit from the interactions with other cultures and be able to serve the health care industry more effectively – and be better able to deal with 9-11 sensitivities.

New Work Options

- Flextime
- Telecommuting
- Job sharing
- Virtual offices

The Work Environment

New Work Options for the Work Environment

"Employers that take steps to offer flexible work programs will be increasingly sought out by employees who need to balance a variety of roles. Pursuing this direction may better position firms to deal with the work force of tomorrow, placing them a step ahead of those who do not."—Kush and Stroh [10]

With the onset of technological growth, new work options have also emerged. More and more organizations are offering alternative work options to their employees to accommodate family needs and geographical constraints and to provide additional benefits. Some of the new work options include:

- Flextime
- Telecommuting
- Job sharing
- Virtual offices

Flextime

Flextime allows an employee to select the hours he or she will work within the practice's operating hours. There are usually specified time limits set by the practice and in most cases, the employee still works the standard number of weekly hours. There are two types of popular flextime arrangements: flex hours and compressed workweeks.

Flex hours allow employees to start and end at various times. For instance, if a practice is open from eight in the morning until six in the evening, employees may start at nine and leave at closing, or start earlier and end earlier. Employees opting for compressed workweeks may work four 10-hour days and have three days off. These arrangements work well for employees with child or adult care issues and who need more time with their families.

This arrangement offers win-win strategies for employees and practices. Flextime can be an added benefit used to attract and retain talent and employees are happier with this work option. For employees who have a long commute, it also limits the amount of time commuting if they opt for a compressed workweek. [11]

Telecommuting

One of the hottest trends in workplaces is telecommuting and many experts predict that it will be the biggest trend of the new century. According to the survey conducted in 2000 by Chicago-based international outplacement firm, Challenger, Gray & Christmas, 43 percent of human resource executives believe that the workforce of the future will be increasingly mobile.[12] In many organizations the Internet and collaborative software applications have made it evident that employees don't have to be in the same building to work closely together. This will not apply to employees in group practices that have direct patient care.

A recent study of 600 employers in the Washington, DC area, found that 37 percent offered a telecommuting program. The survey, conducted by SHRM (Society for Human Resource Management) also stated that 50 percent of organizations with more than 5,000 employees used telecommuting as well as 26 percent of organizations with fewer than 250 employees. These figures reflect a 20 increase from those polled in 1997.[13]

At Winston-Salem, North Carolina-based Novant Health offers job-sharing and telecommuting for jobs that allow it, like medical coding, transcription and billing. The hospital's family-friendly benefits are important to employee retention.[14]

According to the Washington, DC-based International Telework Association and Council (ITAC), teleworkers are more prone to be urban area dwellers rather than live in rural areas or small towns. The Telework America 2000 research survey indicated that teleworking is most common in the manufacturing, business services, construction, banking, insurance, transport and communications industries. However, essentially every industrial sector in the America has teleworkers.[15] Although not yet heavily used in the health care industry, it's possible that some jobs of the future may lend themselves to telecommuting as a work option.

Benefits of Telecommuting

Telecommuting is a great answer to reduce commutes and address employees' needs to care for their families. It also addresses social concerns such as congested highways and pollution. For some organizations, telecommuting broadens their pool of job applicants because it removes geographic boundaries of employees capable of performing quality work from a distance. Other organizations have found that telecommuting also reduces stress in the workplace and that employee productivity is up along with the quality of their work.[16]

Where to Learn More About Telecommuting

Practices interested in learning more about the pros and cons of telecommuting have a variety of resources to explore. The Telecommuting Knowledge Center offers literature, consultants, products and services to support telecommuting. Its online articles cover topics such as how to hire remote workers, employee retention, working at home with children and how to prepare for telecommuting.

SHRM also has telecommuting information on its Web site, some available to the public and some available only to its

160,000 worldwide members. Information offered to members includes "10 tips for managing telecommuters" and a sample telecommunications policy. This sample policy indicates that a meeting should take place between the employee, manager and human resource manager before entering into a telecommuting agreement. The meeting should cover job responsibilities, equipment needs, taxes and legal implications.[17]

MGMA's 2001 book, *Tracking Hot HR Trends*, offers a policy guideline and issues to consider before offering telecommuting or telework options to employees.[18] Other resources also include the American Telecommuting Organization (www.knowledgetree.com) and the International Telework Association and Council (www.telecommute.org).

Job Sharing

Many women and men are faced with the challenge of continuing their careers, raising their families and caring for their elderly parents. Job sharing is becoming a work option that allows employees to continue working while taking care of other personal demands.

Job sharing is a flexible work arrangement where two or more employees share the responsibilities of a full-time position. Although this concept has been used since the early 1980s, it has become more prevalent during the past decade. Primarily used by women with childcare needs, current trends are finding that men are also exploring this work option.

The positions most likely suited for job sharing include information systems, finance, marketing and administration. In the future, more positions may be re-designed to use this work option. Health care organizations have used a form of job sharing for years via part-time and on-call workers,

Benefits to Employees

- Creates a sense of balance between work and personal needs;
- Preserves career skills and status within their industry;
- Maintains practice benefits if part-timers receive them; and
- Allows both career and family goals to be met.

Benefits to Practices

- Acts as a benefit to attract and retain talent;
- Enables new employees to "get up to speed" quicker;
- Perceived as an incentive for many professionals who view time as important as money;
- Increases job satisfaction ; and
- Increases morale and productivity for employees who have a more balanced life—anxiety and stress levels are also lower.

For practices interested in learning more about job sharing, a great resource can be found through Job Sharing Resources, an employment services company located in Long Island, NY. It is dedicated to making job sharing a realistic opportunity for organizations and their employees. This resource can help your practice and its employees locate other interested job sharing contacts. Also, look within your community to locate other resources.[19]

Virtual Offices

"Until recently, when you said you worked with someone, you meant by implication that you worked in the same place for the same organization. Suddenly though, in the blink of an evolutionary eye, people no longer must be co-located—or in the same place—in order to work together. Now, many people work in 'virtual teams' that transcend distance, time zones, and organizational boundaries."—J. Lipnack [20]

Although not an alternative work option used by many practices, there be may opportunities for this concept to work in health care organizations for some positions. Most virtual offices and work teams are linked through technology and allow organizations to have co-workers and teammates that work from their homes. It's telecommuting without commuting.

If your practice has multiple locations in different parts of your area or in other states, virtual offices and work teams may be conducive to your organization. Here are several applications of virtual offices that may be used in the health care industry:

- Scheduling for provider care (answer phones and book appointments)
- Patient service (answer patient calls and questions)
- Ask-a-Nurse (answer calls with medical questions)
- Bookkeeper and accounting services
- Strategic planning team
- Claims office (process claims and handle follow-up with patients and providers)

If your practice is interested in creating virtual offices and work teams, consider how to establish these important variables that can make or break this work option:

- ❑ Trust—Employees from different locations, cultures and technical backgrounds want to know they can rely on other team members and that everyone will make an equal contribution to the practice--whether they are working together in person or apart. Ongoing communication and follow-through are important for team members to develop trust with their "virtual" team members.
- ❑ Interaction--Schedule face-to-face meetings and/or social occasions on a regular basis to ensure that personal relationships develop.
- ❑ Expectations—Without the usual organizational walls to serve as physical boundaries, virtual teams need guidelines to operate effectively. Managing expectations is necessary in this creative work environment to offset frustrations encountered with the system and other team members. Clear definitions of work and performance are important when managers may not be physically present.
- ❑ Cultural differences—These differences exist, even those between departments within the same practice. The lack of cohesion and participation of team members can damage productivity and the ability to work together in the future. Ensure that team members have a good working relationship and that differences are addressed in a timely manner. The practice should offer mediation and conflict resolution training as a tool to help employees discuss issues and reach mutual understanding.

- ❑ Technical coordination—Virtual offices and work teams depend on computer and communication technology to share databases, spreadsheets, and other pertinent information with team members. Check for technical compatibility and ensure that virtual work team members have access to technical help when needed. Coordinate such initiatives through your IT support.

How to Build Alternative Work Options Into Your Practice

If your practice decides that alternative work options would be supported by employees and management, use the following guidelines to explore these options further:

1. Decide which alternative work options your practice would like to offer.
2. Determine which positions are applicable for each option selected.
3. Compare the costs, advantages and disadvantages for each option selected.
4. Hold "stakeholder" meetings with managers, employees and key departments to determine the feasibility of implementing work options effectively.
5. Based on the results of the meetings and the support of the stakeholders, try a couple of pilot demonstrations to see what challenges and solutions arise.
6. If the work options offer viable solutions for employees, managers and the practice, you're on your way to developing a new way of working.

The table presented in Figure 1-2 provides an overview of each of the work options presented, along with possible benefits and challenges for your practice.

Figure 1-2
Alternative Work Options

	Practice Benefits	Practice Challenges
Flextime	• Reduces employee turnover due to personal challenges and commute time. • Added incentive to attract and retain talent. • Opens up an additional talent pool not available previously. • Employees are less stressed and more satisfied.	• Creates different work schedules for employees. • Managers and supervisors have to ensure proper coverage during practice hours. • Potential resentment from other employees.
Telecommuting	• Savings on additional office space. • Reduces employee turnover due to personal challenges and commute time. • Added incentive to attract and retain talent. • Opens up an additional talent pool not available previously. • Employees are less stressed and more satisfied.	• Logistics of coordinating employees off-site. • Technology and compatibility issues. • Feeling included in the rest of the team. • Communication problems. • Lack of face-to-face interaction.
Job Sharing	• Reduces employee turnover due to personal challenges and commute time. • Added incentive to attract and retain talent. • Opens up an additional talent pool not available previously. • Employees are less stressed and more satisfied.	• Maintains different work schedules for employees. • Requires special work plan and tracking of responsibilities. • Communication challenges between job sharing participants and other employees. • Potential resentment from other employees.

Virtual office	• Less stress. • Increased productivity. • Better time management.	• Logistics for offsite offices. • Technology and compatibility issues. • Harder to develop interpersonal relationships with co-workers and customers. • Communication issues.

With so many new work options being introduced successfully in organizations, it's possible that the phrase "going to work" will mean something different for most workers. Work for them will be what they do, not the place they go to do their work.

Summary

Performance Management in the New Century

Since the release of MGMA's *The Medical Practice Performance Management Manual: How to Evaluate Employees* in 1993, there has been a lot of discussion about balanced scorecards, knowledge workers and retaining top talent. All of these topics have a lot in common—an emphasis on the importance of measuring your practice's performance in ways that go beyond traditional reporting systems.

Performance management is not a fad but an approach that continues to be refined by organizations worldwide. Many practices now recognize that non-financial indicators—such as patient satisfaction, and employee morale and turnover—have a major influence on the practice's long-term performance. With the demands for increased service and decreased resources looming on the horizon for the health care industry, performance management becomes even more important.

This book reflects the newest trends, refined best practices and new tools to help practices get the best performance from their employees and to give them a competitive position in the industry.

In this chapter, you explored the changing landscape of the workplace—the new workforce, its diverse challenges and benefits and alternative work options. You also learned that performance management is here to stay and becoming a vital component of most organizations, particularly those in health care.

References:

1. Ron Zemke, Claire Raines and Bob Filipczak, *Generations at Work,* 1999.

2. *The 2001 Employee Review,* Randstad North America, Atlanta, GA, 2001.

3. The Diversity Training Group, www.diversitydtg.com.

4. Mark Van Buren, William Woodwell, Jr., *The 2000 ASTD Trends Report: Staying Ahead of the Winds of Change,* Alexandria, VA, December 2000.

5. Roland Benson, "Cultural Diversity in Health Care is Part of Good Customer Service," South Florida Business Journal, July 1997.

6. Vanessa Weaver and Shawn Coker, "Globalization and Diversity," Mosaics, Society for Human Resource Management, January/February 2001, Vol. 7, No.1.

7. The Diversity Training Group, www.diversitydtg.com.

8. Howard Kim, "Managing Diversity," American Medical News, January 1999.

9. Minnesota Cultural Diversity Center, October 2001 newsletter.

10. Thomas Faulhaber, "Flextime and the Emerging Business," The Business Forum Online, March 3, 1000.

11. Dawn Rosenberg McKay, "An Alternative Work Option: Flextime," www.careerplanning.about.com, 2001.

12. John McHutchion, "Telecommuting Biggest Workplace Trend: Survey," www.canoe.ca/MoneyNewsTechnology, January 2001.

13. Christine Cube, Washington Business Journal, July 6, 2001.

14. Megan Malugani, "Healthcare Benefits Get Progressive," www.medsearch.com.

15. *Telework America 2000 Research Report,* International Telework Association and Council, www.telecommute.org, Washington, D.C.

16. "Telework Works," U.S. Office of Personnel Management, Office of Merit Systems Oversight and Effectiveness. May 2001 Special Study Report.

17. Christine Cube, Washington Business Journal, July 6, 2001.

18. Alys Novak and Courtney Price, *Tracking Hot HR Trends,* Medical Group Management Association, Denver, 2001.

19. www.jobsharing.com, (800) 509-9982.

20. J. Lipnack and J. Stamps, *Virtual Teams: Reaching Across Space, Time, and Organizations with Technology,* Hohn Wiley and Sons, Inc., New York, NY, 1997.

Attracting, Retaining and Developing Top Talent

Chapter 2

Although it's generally the management team that initiates strategic planning and determines organizational goals, performance is mainly achieved through its employees. Some managers and supervisors think it would be easier to achieve high performance if they could just hire "stars." In the book, *Hidden Value: How Great Organizations Achieve Extraordinary Results with Ordinary People,* the authors Charles Reilly and Jeffrey Pfeffer indicate that only 10 percent of the people are going to be in the top 10 percent of the workforce. According to the authors and some of the organizations they interviewed, there aren't enough "stars" to go around. Organizations have to learn how to get better performance from all employees.[1]

Talent management for many organizations continues to be a challenge. When there are low unemployment rates, practices have more difficulty attracting new employees and keeping the ones they already have. The recurring nursing shortage is a good example of the type of challenge facing many health care organizations today. Developing strategies for recruiting and retaining talent is more necessary than before.

In this chapter, we'll explore best practices for attracting, retaining and developing talent for your practice. As staffing shortages and low employment levels continue to be a challenge for health care organizations, it becomes increasingly important to attract and retain the best employees your practice can afford. Beyond your practice's efforts of competing for the best employees, it will need to meet its performance goals by attracting and retaining "good" employees.

"Good" employees have the capability, and can use that capability, to perform in a high-achieving manner to accomplish the goals of the practice. There are good people in all organizations and in every occupation. The level of education and experience are not the only measures your practice uses to define "top talent." All employees bring something unique to your organization. They become even more valuable when led by other good people who develop them into highly productive teams.

When your recruiting efforts for talent are successful, the next objective is to enable the new team member to perform to his or her potential, and to keep that person on the team. This chapter offers many good ideas on getting new employees and keeping them once they are on their way to becoming "stars."

Best Practices for Attracting Top Talent

Practices have a choice: they can either chase the same scarce talent, or decide to focus on a more useful, and much more difficult strategy—building a talent pool that makes it possible for staff to perform like "stars." Take for example the recruiting strategies of PSS World Medical who, from 1996-2001, has enjoyed a growth rate of 52 percent. PSS focuses on finding the right people with the right attitudes and values to fit into its culture. It does hire as many experienced people as possible in sales and operations and usually recruits employees from its competitors.

Recruiting is largely based on personal referrals from PSS staff members and relies more on word-of-mouth scouting than newspaper advertising. PSS has built a successful organization by targeting people who are similar to its culture. PSS employees look for these characteristics during peer interviews and behavior event interviewing with managers:

- Ambitious
- Driven
- Competitive
- Athletic
- Positive attitude
- Self-initiative
- Entrepreneurial

PSS World Medical is not alone in depending on employee referrals for attracting new talent. Some companies provide rewards for employee referrals that lead to new hires. A medical device manufacturing organization in Boulder, CO, offers rewards based on the position, experience and skill level needed. Hard-to-fill positions are rewarded more than those easily filled by ads. One employee received $2,500 for referring two engineers who were hired by his organization.

More and more organizations are relying on multiple recruiting sources to attract good candidates. Some sources work better than others, depending on the medical practice and geographic location. Savvy organizations use a variety of recruiting channels and methods, including:

- In-house recruiters
- Employee referral programs
- Headhunters
- Advertising
- Temporary and permanent staffing agencies
- Campus recruiting
- Internet job boards
- Web site job announcements
- Internal recruiting and promotions

What Attracts Candidates to Your Practice?

In a nationwide survey conducted in 2000 by Watson Wyatt Worldwide, a recognized leader in organizational development, employees were asked what motivates them to accept employment with an organization. Fifteen benefits and workplace characteristics were presented and employees were asked to rate the degree to which each would influence their decision to apply and work for an organization. The top three influences were:

- Compensation—one of the top three factors in three age groups
- Benefits—highest for two age groups, lower for workers under the age of 30
- Opportunity to develop skills—was rated in the top five for all three age groups

Compensation is more than just base pay. Consider using rewards as part of your compensation strategy. Rewards may be monetary and non-monetary. (Results of this study are available through Watson and Wyatt Worldwide or on their Web site at www.watsonwyatt.com.) The following list provides examples of both types of rewards. Chapter 7 focuses on using rewards as part of your performance management system.

Monetary Rewards

✓ Sign-on bonus
✓ Stocks and options
✓ Spot bonus
✓ Retention bonus
✓ Group incentives
✓ Project incentives
✓ Exempt overtime
✓ Skill pay premiums
✓ Comp time off

Non-Monetary Rewards

✓ Advancement opportunities
✓ Flexible work schedules
✓ Opportunities to learn new skills
✓ Career development (non-promotional)
✓ Work-from-home
✓ Reduced work week
✓ Job redesign
✓ Sabbaticals

Tips for Creating Effective Job Postings

- Notice—grab the candidate's attention
- Interest—create appeal in the position
- Longing—build desire to work for your practice
- Act—provide ways for the candidate to respond

Effective Recruiting Starts with the Job Posting

If you advertise for positions, your first impression with candidates is your job posting. Learn to write job ads that attract good candidates by following these tips for creating effective job postings:

Notice—The role of the job posting is to get the potential candidate's attention. Use exciting job titles to generate interest in the position and for candidates to learn more about your opportunity. Example: Wanted: Medical Office Manager Extraordinaire—an Exciting Entrepreneurial Opportunity for the Right Person! The next paragraph explains why this position is an exciting opportunity.

Interest—Create appeal in the position and working for your practice. Describe the details of the position and its requirements. State what the person will be doing daily in this role and the challenges he or she will face. Explain what it's like to work for the practice and how the job will benefit and challenge him or her. List only the job experience and skills that are absolutely necessary. Avoid listing everything on your "wish list." Determine what skills your practice is willing to train on and keep in mind legal requirements for EEO and ADA compliance.

Longing—Build desire for the candidate to work for your practice. List the benefits your practice provides and how working there will improve the candidate's life. Job seekers today are looking for "what's in it for me?" and not just what they can do for you. Some companies mention the pay range for the position in this part of the ad, others don't. Companies have had success doing both, so it's really your preference. Examples of building desire to work for your practice may include:

- Pay that exceeds industry standards
- On-the-job skills training
- Tuition reimbursement
- Flexible work schedule
- Performance bonuses
- Free onsite cafeteria
- Onsite daycare

- Attractive office and great staff
- 401(k) plan

Act—You want the candidate to act after reading the job posting. This is the "call to action" part of the ad. Indicate how the candidate can follow up, including e-mail, online, fax, telephone, snail mail or in person. Don't assume that candidates know how to contact you. Examples of exciting phrases that motivate job seekers to act:

- Don't miss out on this opportunity—Apply Now!
- We're looking forward to reading your resume—Apply Now!
- Take charge of your career—Apply Today!
- Don't Miss Out! You're Going to Love Working with Our Practice! Apply Now!

For more information on attracting top talent, great articles can be found on recruiting web sites. Search for new recruiting sites on the Internet by using a search engine and typing in "attracting" or "recruiting" in the search field and browsing various headhunter and recruiter sites.

Check out these sites that specialize in health care recruiting:

www.globalhealthjobs.com
www.medhunter.com
www.mycomphealthonline.com
www.hcrecruiters.com
www.healthcarejobstore.com

Best Practices for Retaining Top Talent

Once you hire and train new employees, how do you keep them motivated and committed to your practice? When unemployment levels are low, employers face a workforce attrition crisis. Changing workforce demographics, such as the smaller pool of desirable labor (25 – 34 year olds) and the impact of downsizing on employee loyalty can also cause practices to focus more on retaining talented workers.

Health care employees have more choices about where to work than ever before. Job seekers can find openings and information about organizations via the Internet, from trade publications and through professional recruiters. Today's practices rely on their top performers to innovate and provide services that keep patients and attract new ones. Human assets are critical for a practice's survival.

So how does a practice stand out from the crowd to be an "employer-of-choice?" Smart practices understand that workforce needs have changed and become more complex. The employment contract has changed on both sides of employer-employee agreements. Employers still have the same expectations about employees while many employees are uncertain about their work future. It's not a surprise that employee morale is lower and that turnover is higher.

Retention was less of an issue in the past for practices. The unspoken employer/employee contract stated that employees were expected to:

- Work hard;
- Be loyal to the practice; and
- Give the practice their full focus.

And in return, employees received:

- Lifetime employment;
- A "family" atmosphere; and
- Regular raises and promotions.

Employee attrition is costly and impacts your practice both financially and operationally. The cost of replacing an employee—advertising, interviewing, training and other staff members' time—can easily be double that of the departing employee's salary. Other hidden costs such as the loss of patient relationships and stress can send a message that the practice is unstable.

Some employee attrition is inevitable, and even may be desirable so a practice can add new talent and skills to its pool. For many practices, the highest attrition occurs with employees who are compensated the least (e.g., receptionists, nurse aides, lab technicians).

As a result of nationwide retention studies conducted by Watson Wyatt Worldwide from 1997 to 2000, results have determined a positive correlation between organizational success and a culture that promotes employee involvement, two-way communication and opportunities for advancement. Seven specific factors have been determined to influence employee commitment with trust in leadership and the chance to use skills coming in at the top:

Trust in leadership–Employees who have high trust and confidence with their senior management stay the longest. Trust in the eyes of employees means:

- Promoting qualified employees;
- Gaining support for business decisions from employees;
- Motivating employees to perform at high levels; and
- Explaining rationale behind major business decisions.

Chance to use skills on the job—Employees want to use what they know and have a chance to develop new skills. There are several ways to enhance employee skills, including:

- Create self-directed work teams that promote personal leadership and a rotation of team roles.
- Work with employees to determine their career goals, identify new skills to be developed, and create opportunities to obtain and use these new skills.
- Recognize that employees have skill sets not utilized in their current roles and take the time to learn more about them than just their jobs.

Job security—Although organizations can no longer guarantee lifetime employment, they can work with employees to be "lifetime employable." Sharing information about organization goals, involving employees in decision-making, and developing "contracts" for accountability helps employees to realize their role in creating a financially viable organization.

Competitive Rewards—Many organizations underestimate the power of strategic rewards. In a recent study on the use of rewards, only 24 percent of employers polled thought of rewards as a way to engage employees in improving their performance. Employees consider recognition and rewards to be additional perks.

Quality of organization's products and services—Employees want to work for an organization they are proud of. They want to feel part of a larger entity than themselves. Involving employees in giving and receiving feedback lets them know the organization values their input in creating quality products and services.

Lower levels of work-related stress—No job is without stress and today's employees are more concerned about balancing their work and personal lives. Employees appreciate when organizations acknowledge that they have family obligations and a need for recreation.

Organization honesty and integrity—Employees who feel they have to compromise on their personal integrity won't stay with their employer long. Managers need to "walk their talk" and be role models in operational practices. Showing genuine concern for employees and customers, as well as delivering on promises is important in developing employee commitment.

Other factors—Several other factors play a role in retaining talent. Although a few of them reflect some overlap in the seven factors just mentioned, it's worth drawing attention to them. Organizations with higher employee retention rates:

- Treat employees well and fairly.
- Practice flexibility in benefit plans and work hours.
- Promote employees to self-manage their career paths.
- Communicate openly with employees about the business—goals, challenges and changes.
- Offer training, tuition reimbursement and other ways for employees to develop and enhance their career skills.

Keep in mind that "one size doesn't fit all" and not all employees want the same things. Mature workers and baby-boomers are more interested in job stability, benefits and a "family" atmosphere. Younger generational workers like Gen Xers and Gen Yers prefer skills development, flexibility and incentives.

Consider developing a flex-benefit plan that allows employees to choose their benefits based on their values and needs. Working mothers, for instance, are becoming increasingly interested in getting childcare assistance. Section 125 plans that provide a "cafeteria-style" approach to benefits allow employees to set aside pre-tax income for childcare and medical expenses. You may even offer a menu of holidays from which employees can select based on the number of days allotted.

Best Practices for Developing Top Talent

For employees to perform at peak performance they need opportunities to grow. There are many different ways to develop top talent, including special projects, seminars, job enrichment and personal coaching. Employees want to grow professionally and learn new skills. In today's job market, it isn't enough to retain employees; your practice should also help develop them.

As part of the performance management process, managers and supervisors discuss developmental needs with employees and together, create an action plan with objectives to address them. These objectives can be a part of the employee's individual performance plan. Designing an individual development plan with each employee enhances his or her feeling of importance—both for self-esteem and significance within the organization.

For example, as a result of Susan's performance review, she agrees with her supervisor that she should enhance her listening skills to be more emphatic to senior patients. She and her supervisor discuss courses that are available at a nearby community college. Susan will contact the college to register for the next semester.

After discussing development plans with employees, managers and supervisors should document agreed outcomes by:

- Writing down the specific steps to be taken for each developmental area;
- Indicating the names of any people who will assist the employee;

- Stating end dates of the completion of the plan's objectives; and
- Indicating how successful completion of the plan's objectives will be appraised.

By providing a positive learning culture, you can motivate employees to apply their talents and expertise to help your practice and their careers. Consider these other ideas your practice can use to develop top talent:

- Give employees new challenging responsibilities.
- Cross-train employees to learn new jobs and skills.
- Provide financial support to employees interested in continuing their formal education.
- Send employees to seminars to enhance or learn new skills.
- Allow employees to explore memberships in trade and professional associations to meet, interact and learn from other professionals.
- Have employees train others in areas they have strength or expertise.
- Offer learning materials for personal and professional growth by establishing a library of books, audiotapes, videos and periodicals on a variety of job-related and non-job related topics.
- Encourage employees to borrow learning materials from local libraries.
- Contact local bookstores located near your practice to inquire about new books on topics of interest to your employees.

Summary

Changing for the Future

Changing recruiting and retaining strategies is comfortable for some practices and not for others. Practices that use creative and different ways to recruit, retain and develop talent are on their way to being the "employers of choice" with tomorrow's health care workers. By following many of the ideas offered in this chapter, not only will your practice retain its "stars," it will also attract more high-quality employees.

References:

1. Charles Reilly and Jeffrey Pfeffer, *Hidden Value: How Great Organizations Achieve Extraordinary Results with Ordinary People,* Harvard Business School Press, 2000.

2. CIO, September 15, 2000, pp. 226-246.

Information collected about attracting, retaining and developing talent came from various sources, including the following:

www.vault.com
www.hr.com
www.shrm.org

The New Bottom Line: Performance Management

Chapter 3

Many practices may lose performance because they don't really understand what performance management is. Is it safe to assume that if all employees are getting satisfactory performance reviews annually from their supervisors, then the practice must be doing well? Maybe not. If the performance of the employee, or unit or department, does not directly contribute to organizational results, chances are the medical practice is not performing well. And the employees aren't performing well either. Be assured—everyone's working hard; doing certain things right—but they may not be doing the right things or working smart.

Performance management is a way to ensure that the practice gets results from all employees, regardless of their position or tenure. It's more than job descriptions that simply list job duties and responsibilities. Job descriptions usually don't tell employees what specific results are expected of them. They are not a tool to show the manager or supervisor how well employees are doing at their jobs. And performance evaluations—that's just paperwork for many supervisors and employees, something required by management.

Performance management is a broader approach to managing employee performance. This chapter explains the difference between a performance management process and system, and identifies the six most common challenges.

A Successful Performance Management Process

1. Organizational goals and objectives
2. Individual performance planning
3. Employee performance measurements
4. Ongoing feedback and coaching
5. Performance reviews
6. Recognition and rewards

What is a Performance Management Process?

In MGMA's classic reference, *The Medical Practice Performance Management Manual: How to Evaluate Employees,*[1] a performance management process is described as, "the idea of constant communication throughout the work year rather than a once-a-year discrete event." An effective performance management process is more than just performance evaluations. It's an integrated process that's designed to improve the way that work gets done. It emphasizes helping employees perform their jobs in ways that align with the organization's plans. A performance management process is successful when outcomes are tied to staff performance.

The HR literature and case studies clearly show that organizations which implement and use a good performance management process perform better financially and non-financially than organizations that do not value performance measurement.

A successful performance management process encompasses these six components:

- Organizational goals and objectives;
- Individual performance planning;
- Employee performance measurements;
- Performance reviews;
- Ongoing feedback and coaching; and
- Recognition and rewards.

Organizational Goals and Objectives

It's essential that a group practice have clear strategic goals and objectives. This provides the context for performance management so that individual performance is aligned with the organization's overall goals. It's important that employees know their roles play an important part in the practice achieving its goals and that everyone affects outcomes.

A group practice has to achieve certain objectives to be successful. For instance, the organization may determine that "providing quality care" is an important objective. If the practice meets this objective, its patients will be satisfied with their care and the practice will continue to thrive.

Samples of organizational goals include:

- Provide excellent medical care to all patients.
- Develop and reward a quality workforce.
- Maintain effective operating procedures.
- Create a positive work environment where team members help one another to meet patients' needs.

Examples of organizational objectives:

- The practice responds to patient concerns in an efficient and timely manner.
- Patient care surveys indicate that the service received is excellent or above average.
- Patients receive adequate information from their health care provider.
- Claims processing is efficient and patient complaints are low.
- Employees receive ongoing skills training and are rewarded for excellent performance.
- Procedures are documented, understood by staff members and followed.

When organizational goals and objectives are clearly stated, individual performance plans can then be created.

Individual Performance Planning

Employees at all levels of the organization should have clearly defined goals and objectives that directly link to those of the organization. Both the manager and the employee should meet to define how performance is to be planned and evaluated. By making the employee a "customer" of the process, managers and employees are on the same side. (For information on individual and employee performance see Chapter 4.)

Employee Performance Measurements

New thinking in the areas of performance management reflects an emphasis on connecting employee behavior to the organization's goals. The most effective performance management process collects, analyzes and distributes information about how well employees are meeting its goals. Reports should include preventive and corrective actions to increase employee performance. (Review Chapter 4 for more information on performance measurements.)

Performance Reviews

Actual performance is reviewed periodically to offer employees feedback and preventive and/or corrective action to keep them on track in meeting their objectives. Performance reviews should focus on performance results, pinpoint specific issues and problems and offer corrective action. Effective performance reviews are two-way discussions and written documentation focusing on employee performance: areas of excellence, improvement goals, developmental needs and action plans. (See Chapter 4 for best practices in performance reviews.)

Ongoing Feedback and Coaching

Communication between managers and employees throughout the year ensure that problems are identified early and intervention is part of the process. Managers provide feedback about performance on a regular basis. Coaching is an ongoing process of communication focused on improving current performance and building skills for the future. Coaching may be informal conversation or notes, as well as formal methods that consist of coaching meetings and written documentation. By engaging in this kind of consistent dialogue, there are no surprises during annual performance appraisals. (Chapters 3 and 4 have detailed information on coaching and feedback.)

Recognition and Rewards

Employees want and need recognition. Without it, many of them feel undervalued or not appreciated. Recognizing and rewarding positive behavior and performance is a way to initiate change in organizations. Overall, employees respond favorably, are more motivated, exceed job expectations, and stay with an organization when they feel their contributions are valued.

Recognition and rewards do not have to be monetary to be effective. With a shift toward variable pay and other nontraditional reward systems, organizations have found multiple ways to thank employees for doing a good job. Some employees prefer comp time, a handwritten note, or praise during team meetings. Pay attention to what employees want and need and then look for ways to reward them. Recognition and rewards say, "We value your contribution and care about your well-being." (Best practices for rewards and recognition are highlighted in Chapter 5.)

Figure 3.1 provides an overview of a performance management process. This model can work in all practices, regardless of its size. Employees want to know what's expected of them, how they're performing and expect to be evaluated fairly, and recognized for good performance. The most effective processes are done consistently so employees know what to expect and don't feel that it's another "program for the quarter."

Figure 3.1
Performance Management Process

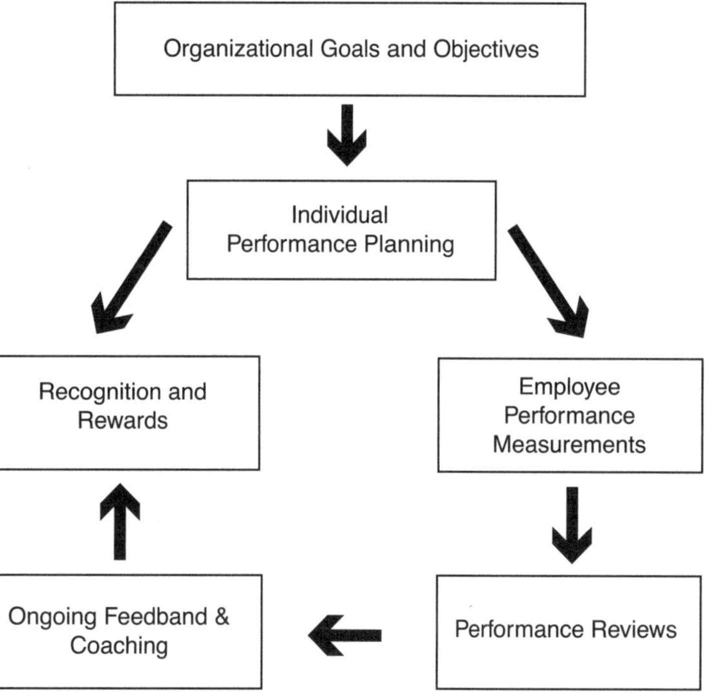
Organizational Goals and Objectives
Individual Performance Planning
Recognition and Rewards
Employee Performance Measurements
Ongoing Feedband & Coaching
Performance Reviews

Performance Management System Strategies

A performance management system incorporates different tools and processes that allow an organization to identify and achieve the goals of its business. It's a different type of management system whose primary purpose is to enable an organization and its employees to achieve greater levels of effectiveness and connectedness.

A performance management process is "how" employee performance is evaluated in an organization. It integrates the separate components of a performance management system and indicates how each component interacts with the others.

Basically, a performance management system is a way to get results from employees. The most successful systems link employee performance to the organization's outcomes. There are four areas, or pillars, of an effective performance management system that must exist for successful implementation:

- ✓ **Specified Results**—Clearly stated goals that individuals on all levels understand and clearly indicate what's needed to achieve them.
- ✓ **Reliable Measurement**—Defined and tracked results that impact individual and organization performance.
- ✓ **Performance Standards**—Mutually agreed upon criteria, used to describe how well an individual must perform.
- ✓ **Effective Consequences**—Ways to recognize, reward and retain top performers in the organization.[2]

Assess Your Organization's Performance Strategies

How does your organization rate on performance strategies? Assess your current performance strategies by responding to the following Group Practice Performance Strategies Rating. Select only one response for each statement. The right answers are listed at the bottom of the assessment.

Group Practice Performance Strategies Rating
(Select all that apply)

PART I. Indicate how often your practice measures performance.

1. **We set specific, measurable and ongoing performance goals:**
   ___ A. Never.
   ___ B. Sometimes.
   ___ C. Often
   ___ D. Always.

2. **We recognize staff for exceptional performance:**
   ___ A. Never.
   ___ B. Sometimes.
   ___ C. Often
   ___ D. Always.

3. **We reward staff for exceptional performance:**
   ___ A. Never.
   ___ B. Sometimes.
   ___ C. Often
   ___ D. Always.

4. **As part of the management team, I receive:**
   ___ A. Feedback on my performance on a regular basis.
   ___ B. Performance feedback during my annual review.
   ___ C. Feedback daily.
   ___ D. No feedback which means "I'm doing okay, otherwise I'd hear about it."

Part I Score: Your practice earns one point for each best practice answers—1D, 2D and 3D and 4A. Continue with Part II.

PART II. Indicate how your medical practice measures performance.

1. **We set specific, measurable and ongoing performance goals:**
   ___ A. For the practice, but not for individual employees.
   ___ B. For the practice, but only for managers and supervisors.
   ___ C. For the practice and for all employees, including physicians and patient providers.
   ___ D. We don't set specific, measurable and ongoing performance goals.

2. **We recognize and reward staff consistently:**
   ___ A. For positive behaviors only.
   ___ B. For both performance results and positive behaviors.
   ___ C. For longevity of employment
   ___ D. For attendance.
   ___ E. We don't recognize and reward consistently.

3. **We reward performance by:**
   ___ A. Selecting and honoring an employee of the month.
   ___ B. Giving everyone on the team recognition or a reward.
   ___ C. Celebrating the person who had the best attendance record, who is the most liked by patients, etc.
   ___ D. Acknowledging everyone who reached a predetermined performance goal.

4. **When we want to make changes to improve our practice's performance, we ask:**
   ___ A. Employees who work with patients daily for advice.
   ___ B. Patients for feedback.
   ___ C. Managers and physicians to get buy-in from the top.
   ___ D. We ask everyone for feedback.

5. **For measuring individual and organization performance, we:**
   ___ A. Don't measure.
   ___ B. Meet with management staff for input.
   ___ C. Meet with all employees including supervisors, managers, physicians, and patient care providers.
   ___ D. Only measure financial performance related to the bottom line (e.g., revenue, ROI, accounts receivables, expenses).

Part II Score: Your practice earns one point for each of these correct answers—1C, 2B, 3D, 4D, 5C. If your total score was 7 or higher, your practice has good performance management strategies. If your score were lower than 7, the subsequent chapters will help you improve your performance management strategies.

The Five Common Challenges with Performance Management Systems:

1. Establishing a consistent structure for responsibility
2. Balancing long-term and short-term focus
3. Focusing on too many measurement factors
4. Tying compensation to performance-driven behavior
5. Implementation of the performance management process is too difficult

Performance Management System Challenges and How to Overcome Them

Although it clearly pays off to install a performance management system, it isn't usually a smooth ride for organizations. These are the five most common challenges with performance management systems:

Challenge 1: Establishing a consistent structure for responsibility

For many practices, there is the challenge of providing consistency and alignment. The market, regulations and technology keep changing. But employees need consistent performance and support from management to develop trust in the performance management system. The management philosophy for your practice must be used consistently by all managers and supervisors for a performance management system to be effective.

Solution: Trust in an organization starts with management actions and behavior. The roles and responsibilities of each management level must be clear and there should be a consistent management style throughout the practice. Doing the right things at the right time is everyone's job. If supervisors/managers don't "walk the talk," the rest of the staff follows suit. Managers and supervisors can support the performance management process and "walk the talk" by being responsible for their own performance goals and ensuring that each employee's performance plan is aligned with the practice's overall goals.

Challenge 2: Balancing long-term and short-term focus

Although some group practices have strategic goals, most focus either on the "big picture" or are too consumed with the "small details." Being disciplined to balance between these two perspectives can be difficult. Translating strategic goals into short-term, measurable action plans seems to be the root cause for this challenge.[3]

Solution: Practices should transfer their strategic goals into short-term action plans that can be measured by managers and employees. The goals are set at the top level of management and action plans are implemented at the staff level. An action plan allows managers and supervisors to communicate the practice's strategic goals in operational terms to employees. In this way, employees can see how their job objectives are linked to the practice's goals.

It may be helpful to define the difference between goals and objectives: Goals are broad targets, generally qualitative rather than quantitative, and are concerned with where the practice is headed. Objectives, on the other hand, are more specific targets that are concerned with how to achieve goals. The key to setting successful action plans is to construct them so that progress towards them is measurable.

For an action plan to be successful, objectives should contain the following elements found in this acronym SMARTER:

S – specific
M – measurement
A – action
R – resources
T – time limit
E – evaluation
R - results

Here are two examples of a medical group practice transferring their strategic goals into short-term, measurable action plans:

A Strategic Goal for a Medical Practice: Provide excellent medical care to all patients.

The Admission Department's Action Plan:

Specific Objective 1: Reduce the average amount of time for patients to be registered from 25 minutes to less than 20 minutes and do so within 30 days.

Measurement: Maintain daily logs indicating the time patients arrive and the actual time patients are registered. Log information will be collected and entered into a database or spreadsheet for analysis.

Resources: None needed. Current staff will log information as needed and enter information collected.

Time Limit: Log information will be maintained for 30 days and reviewed weekly.

Evaluation: Log information will be reviewed weekly and discussed in staff meetings

Results: Log results will be tabulated each week and suggestions from staff meetings will be implemented the following week. An analysis of the month with additional recommendations will be submitted to management.

Specific Objective 2: Increase the accuracy rate of billing information collected during registration from 90 to 95 percent within 60 days.

Measurement: Maintain a log of all registrations and indicate which ones have billing information errors. Enter information into a database or spreadsheet and calculate accuracy ratios.

Resources: None needed. Current accounts receivable staff will log information as needed and enter information collected.

Time Limit: Log information will be maintained for 60 days and reviewed weekly.

Evaluation: Log information will be reviewed weekly and discussed in staff meetings. Determine billing information areas that have the most errors and its causes.

Results: Log results will be tabulated each week and suggestions from staff meetings will be implemented the following week. An analysis of each month with additional recommendations will be submitted to management.

After completing an action plan for the department, managers and supervisors can then work with each employee to develop an individual action plan as part of his or her performance goals.

Challenge 3: Focusing on too many measurement factors

Managers can't measure everything employees are doing. It's important to set specific performance targets for the department, unit or practice and focus on exceptions, analysis and actions. Having too many measurements is cumbersome for the staff and managers who have to collect and disseminate information. Detailed accounts aren't as important as the outcomes.

Solution: Determine which performance measurements are truly important to your practice and which aren't. Select up to four measurement factors that will be used to evaluate performance. Discuss the best way to collect and disseminate information based on your practice's resources. Use performance reviews to evaluate individual progress and create individual action plans with follow-up and evaluation.

Challenge 4: Tying compensation to performance-driven behavior.

Individual compensation should be tied to performance, which is aligned with meeting organizational goals. Many organizations offer a flat salary or hourly wage and do not offer performance pay. Best performers may be compensated the same as others if pay is based on tenure, position and a cost-of-living increase. There is no motivation for meeting individual or organizational goals or improving performance.

Solution: One approach is using a competency pay plan. Each employee has performance standards and receives additional compensation if these standards are met. Performance standards are based on meeting strategic goals and practice- or position-specific objectives. Best performers are recognized and rewarded for their outstanding contributions. The practice also wins by meeting its financial and non-financial expectations.

Example of Competency-Based Pay:

A mid-size clinic has "Focus on Patients" as one its competency areas and rewards employees that meet performance standards for this model. Top performers at the clinic consistently exhibit this set of behaviors:

- Demonstrates a deep understanding of internal customers and patients and their needs.
- Mobilizes the appropriate resources to respond to co-worker and patient needs.
- Takes personal responsibility for co-worker and patient satisfaction.
- Builds credibility and trust with co-workers and patients through open and direct communication (e.g., uses effective listening skills, provides timely feedback)
- Ensures that co-workers and patients believe their issues are given the highest priority.

During performance reviews, employees are rated in each competency area based on a multi-rating system. Top performers are provided bonuses or incentive pay after each review. (For more information on performance-based pay plans, see Chapter 6.)

Challenge 5: Implementation of the performance management process is too difficult

In many organizations, managers and employees don't follow performance management processes because they are complex, burdensome paper trails, and measurements don't accurately reflect performance. After a while, people consider it a waste of time and stop doing it all together.

Solution: Performance management processes need to fit neatly together, be simple to use and follow, and reliable. Have managers and employees meet and discuss how their particular department or unit performance helps meet the practice's overall goals. Agree on overall performance measures and how individual performance should be measured. When implementing a new performance management process, meet quarterly initially and talk about what's working and not working. Thereafter, hold meetings annually to refine its components. Having ongoing feedback between managers and employees is the key to having a performance management system that works and is used by all.

Summary

The Importance of Learning Best Practices from Other Organizations

An old saying goes something like this, "A wise man learns from others' mistakes, a fool by his own." Many physicians and administrators think their practices and work environments are too unique to "model" what others are doing. Although most research in performance management has been around retail, manufacturing and non-health care industries, there is much to gleam from their successes and much of it can be applied to medical practices.

In the chapters to follow, best practice examples will be provided to illustrate how other organizations successfully implement performance management systems. Every practice can utilize performance management to set goals, measure what's important, provide feedback, and create positive consequences for all staff members. Use this resource to develop a system that works for your organization.

References

1 Courtney Price and Alys Novak, *The Medical Practice Performance Management Manual: How to Evaluate Employees,* MGMA, Englewood, CO, 1993.

2 Aubrey Daniels, Ph.D., *Bringing Out the Best in People,* McGraw-Hill Professional Publishing, 1999

3 Andre A. de Waal, *Power of Performance Management,* New York, NY: John Wiley & Sons, 2001

Performance Management Trends

Chapter 4

"Continuous white water" is a term that could be used to describe the overall health care industry. Constant changes in managed care, state and federal requirements, and medical procedures are challenging not only for the best physicians, nurses and hospitals; but also are an ongoing challenge for all health care workers.

In the midst of constant change and chaos, it's important for employees to practice self-management when it comes to their careers. What is "*self-management?*" In the book, *We Are All Self-Employed*, C.S. Hakim explains that all "employees are responsible for working with the organization and the customer and for attending to his or her own personal and professional development."[1]

Employees will practice self-management if they recognize they ARE the CEO of their own careers. Regardless of the economy, the employees should have ownership of their careers and professional development. This is one of the most significant changes in the area of performance management—*empowering employees to self-manage their careers and performance.*

This chapter explores new trends in performance management. Most of these trends focus on helping employees develop self-management skills and accountability to improve performance, and on developing managers and supervisors as coaches and mentors.

The Role of Employees in Performance Management

For many organizations, performance is achieved through people—by what they know, what they can do, and how willing they are to do it. People also need the systems and processes that enable them to reach strategic goals. Managing change, building effective teams, delivering top-notch patient service, and ensuring innovation and creativity can't happen without employees. They are the heart of performance management—without people, whose performance is being measured?

Performance management defines what employees should be doing. It provides ongoing communication between managers and employees throughout the year, links individual performance to organizational goals, and evaluates and rewards good performance.

Characteristics of self-managing employees

What do we know about employees who want to manage their careers and performance? According to Healthcare Dynamics, an organizational development company in Brunswick, ME, that provides leadership and communication training to health care professionals, self-managing employees are more likely to be:

- Clear about their purpose and their direction.
- Aware of their skills and areas for improvement.
- Open to change and willing to accept new challenges.
- Continuously learning to stay ahead in their field and to be marketable.

Employee Performance Development

Performance development gives employees a process of setting goals that are specific to their positions and a way to keep score of their accomplishments. Throughout the performance management process, employees know what's expected from them, how their performance is measured, and how well they meet their performance goals.

Before employees can manage their performance development, they should "begin with the end in mind," or have a clear understanding of the expected outcomes. As Yogi Berra said, "If you don't know where you're going, you may not get there!" An effective performance management process allows employees to be partners in:

- Creating goals and objectives for their specific position.
- Determining performance standards and measurements.
- Receiving regular performance reviews and feedback on how they are meeting agreed-upon expectations.
- Ongoing coaching and feedback opportunities.
- Recognizing and rewarding their accomplishments.
- Managing a career development plan that supports them and the organization.

The Symbiotic Relationship Between Career Management and Performance Development

High potential employees see career development as more important than promotions. Even marginal employees understand how their present performance affects future career opportunities. By linking career management with performance development, employees learn how to align their personal goals with their organization's goals.

A good reflection of how career management and performance management go hand-in-hand is the explanation by Dr. Gerald Sturman, co-author of *Coaching Careers and Performance,* "Career and performance management is the process in which employees take responsibility for developing their ability to make an expanded contribution to the organization...a contribution linking individual work satisfaction to the goals and challenges of the organization."[2]

Job performance is generally black or white. As a manager, your role is to observe, collect feedback from others, and evaluate employee performance. Either the employee is meeting performance standards or not. You provide feedback for improvement and help employees to be successful in their positions.

Career development and coaching, on the other hand, is non-positional. Helping employees manage their careers involves providing a safe venue for employees to discuss their ambitions and supporting them in taking steps to be closer to meeting their individual goals. By practicing effective career and performance coaching, managers gain personal satisfaction and a reputation for being a manager who supports and develops people. This creates value-added advantages for organizations that want to attract and retain talent.[3]

Creating a Symbiotic Relationship in Your Practice

Start with learning about each employee's career goals. Recognize that career development can be frustrating to employees. Career ideals and the reality of job opportunities don't always match. The frustration that employees feel is not just the disparity between the ideal and the real, but the feeling of disempowerment that can come from feeling like the "little fish in the big pond." Sometimes they feel as if there is nothing they can do to get ahead.

Keep in mind that *job performance* is what your employees are doing for a living right now. Career development is more than that—it's the very nature of what people are—their hopes, dreams and ambitions. When employees are satisfied with their job performance, they're more satisfied with the rest of their lives. If more attention is placed on career development, it's possible to improve job performance. This provides a win-win opportunity for organizations and their employees because employee development is also organization development.

Five Elements of Career Management

1. Assessment
2. Investigate
3. Match
4. Choose
5. Manage

Elements of Career Management

Five elements of career management have been identified. Use these elements as a guide during your career management meeting with an employee:

1. **Assessment**—The career management process begins with employees exploring as much about themselves as possible. Help the employee to create an overall vision of his or her work life and determine his or her contribution to the practice:

    - What skills does he or she have that are useful to the practice?
    - What does he or she like about his or her current position?
    - What qualities does he or she possess?
    - What are his or her strengths and weaknesses?

There are many tools available in the market to support managers and employees in doing a career or skills assessment. From do-it-yourself books to online assessments, there is a wealth of resources. Two great do-it-yourself books are, *Managing Your Career with Power,* from the Career Development Team[4] and the most popular book for career development, *What Color is Your Parachute?* by Richard Nelson Bolles.[5]

Managing Your Career with Power focuses on exploring your career options with your current employer, while *What Color is Your Parachute?* concentrates on changing careers or transferring skill sets. Employees interested in online assessments can find great tools at such websites like www.careerstorm.com.

2. **Investigation**—The second element involves research on the part of the employee or with your assistance. Discovering what the challenges, needs and opportunities are within the organization helps the employee to create an internal career map. If your group practice is large, this investigation may include discussions with other departments or divisions.

3. **Matching**—Help the employee to see how his or her assessment aligns with the needs, challenges and opportunities of the practice.

4. **Choosing**—Assist the employee to create short-term and long-term development targets to enhance his or her skills and to excel in his or her current position and to

prepare long-term career goals. No job lasts forever any more, so "what next" must always be considered.

5. **Managing**—After you and the employee have identified a career development plan, discuss specific actions and deadlines to meet for his or her plan on stay on track.

Once you have helped your employees through these elements, you've created the groundwork for them to continue managing their career development. Now they can focus on managing their performance with each position they hold. They also realize what it will take for them to achieve their career goals.

Employee Performance Development

As part of a performance management process, managers meet with employees to discuss individual performance goals. A good rule of thumb is to set annual goals for each employee. In addition to setting goals, managers and employees should agree upon performance standards. While job descriptions identify essential functions and tasks to be done, performance standards define how well each function or task should be performed for employees to meet or exceed expectations.

In *The Medical Practice Performance Management Manual: How to Evaluate Employees,* an evaluation method called BARS (Behaviorally Anchored Rating Scale) is used to establish performance standards.[6] Each function should have specific standard descriptions that explain the differences between Exceeding Expectations, Meeting Expectations, and so forth. Review this tool to see how it would work for you.

Although employees receive periodic reviews where managers and peers evaluate their performance results, it's important for employees to manage and evaluate themselves. A self-evaluation encourages employees to manage their own performance. A sample self-appraisal worksheet is included in *The Medical Practice Performance Management Manual: How to Evaluate Employees.*

In some practices, performance development is offered as a two-part process: An employee uses the self-assessment to generally evaluate his or her performance and the manager also completes an assessment on the employee's performance. During the performance review a comparison is made between the two and differences are discussed.

In other practices, an employee uses a self-evaluation to rate his or her accomplishments in each functional area and presents it to his or her manager as part of the performance review. Ideally, both types of self-evaluations should be completed prior to performance reviews.

A newer trend in self-evaluation is represented in Figure 4-1. Managers and employees determine key function areas to be evaluated, including general core strategies of the practice as well as job-specific competencies. This model allows an employee to reflect on how he or she exhibited or implemented specific performance standards. It also includes a personal development plan for each functional area so he or she can determine appropriate action steps to enhance the competency. Self-evaluations serve as a consistent means for employees to manage their own performance as part of their career development plan.[7]

The first edition of this manual includes a sample self-appraisal worksheet that is worth reviewing (see p. 99).

Figure 4-1

Self-Evaluation Plan

Quality Patient Care

- Listens carefully and responds to patient requests and concerns.
- Delivers friendly, courteous service to internal customers and patients.
- Demonstrates a commitment to increasing patient satisfaction.
- Looks for and makes continuous improvements.
- Performs with accuracy, thoroughness and effectiveness.

I exhibit positive performance in this area by:

I can improve in this area by:

Rating:

___	Well Above	My performance is consistently above expectations.
___	Above	My performance is sometimes above expectations.
___	Meets	My performance meets expectations.
___	Below	My performance is sometimes below expectations.
___	Well Below	My performance is consistently below expectations.

Training and development needed in this area:

Knowledge/Skill	Level of Proficiency Required	Complete By

Focus on Results

- Sets goals in alignment with the group practice's objectives.
- Organizes work to achieve individual goals.
- Identifies and solves problems that come up.
- Achieves targeted results as planned.
- Accomplishes agreed-upon responsibilities.
- Accepts responsibility for his or her own actions.
- Attends work consistently as scheduled.

How I exhibit positive performance in this area:

How I can improve in this area:

Rating:

___ Well Above	My performance is consistently above expectations.
___ Above	My performance is sometimes above expectations.
___ Meets	My performance meets expectations.
___ Below	My performance is sometimes below expectations.
___ Well Below	My performance is consistently below expectations.

Additional section for managers/supervisors

- Implements and follows through with performance management processes.
- Sets clear goals and performance expectations with employees.
- Gives feedback in a respectful and positively constructive way.
- Encourages employees to seek feedback from more than one source.
- Promotes self-development and responsiveness to others' feedback.
- Uses coaching skills effectively to improve employee performance.
- Conducts timely and effective performance reviews.
- Recognizes excellent performance in employees.
- Encourages employees to engage in different learning and development opportunities.

How I exhibit positive performance in this area:

How I can improve in this area:

Rating:

___ Well Above	My performance is consistently above expectations.
___ Above	My performance is sometimes above expectations.
___ Meets	My performance meets expectations.
___ Below	My performance is sometimes below expectations.
___ Well Below	My performance is consistently below expectations.

By providing career and performance development tools, managers help employees to plan and manage their work lives. It also helps employees to become attuned to new work and organizational realities, which includes the need to upgrade their skills to meet future requirements. And rather than waiting for their managers to provide constant direction, employees learn to take responsibility for planning and managing their own careers and performance.

Coaching for Performance

Personal coaching is a hot topic these days and references to coaching are everywhere: people touting the need for a career coach, life coach, transition coach, etc. Why are managers naturally inclined to be good coaching candidates? People have always looked first to their managers for career advice and for support in their professional development.

Coaching is quickly becoming the most popular tool for employee development because: (1) The global economy requires organizations to do more with fewer resources, creating a push for improved employee performance; (2) organizations realize that a one-size-fits-all approach to learning is ineffective. Coaching recognizes individual needs and utilizes a one-on-one development approach; and (3) people in leadership roles are expected to help develop other leaders as part of a recruiting and retention strategy. [8]

What is Performance Coaching?

Performance coaching is "the process by which employees gain the skills, abilities and knowledge they need to develop themselves professionally and become more effective in their jobs."[9] Using performance coaching as a development tool is becoming increasingly popular as managers realize that by coaching effectively, they can increase the performance in employee's current jobs and enhance their potential to do more in future roles.

Performance coaching:

- Clarifies what employees should do and the best ways to do them (otherwise known as "instruction").
- Offers positive reinforcement for good work (another way of looking at "praise").
- Finds ways to redesign employee functions and increase their commitment (what used to be called "empowerment" or "shared leadership").

There are many benefits of using performance coaching. Increased employee performance may be enough for some managers, but consider these benefits as added bonuses if you incorporate coaching as part of your performance management process:

- Your employees require less supervision by you.
- You and your employees no longer have "surprises" during performance reviews.
- You develop better rapport with your employees.
- You are recognized by upper management as having strong "people skills."
- Your department or organization runs smoother than ever before.

Five Performance Coaching Principles

1. Gather information.
2. Listen.
3. Be aware of the environment.
4. Provide instruction.
5. Give feedback.

How to Be a Coach

Coaching employees is a lot like coaching athletes. Great coaches share the same philosophies about their role. Managers who use performance coaching effectively have come to understand these five important principles of coaching:

1. **Gather information**—A good coach knows how to learn as much as possible from an employee without making that person feel as if he or she is being interrogated. Information gathering is important to making sound management decisions.

2. **Listen**—It's not enough to ask the right questions. Good coaches know how to listen with a "third ear" and pay attention to non-verbal as well as verbal messages. They also use their own body language to communicate with employees to let them know they are being heard.

3. **Be aware of the environment**—Coaches talk frequently to employees to measure morale and to look for signs of distress in the workplace that could impact performance.

4. **Provide instruction**—A good coach trains employees individually or in groups to help them perform tasks better. Coaches often spend time assessing the needs of each employee and finding ways to enhance his or her skills.

5. **Give feedback**—Effective coaches know how important feedback is to improve performance. Positive and corrective feedback reinforces the right behaviors and has a direct impact on employee performance.[10]

How Are Your Coaching Skills?

Assess your current coaching skills and discover where you can make some improvements. Indicate your response to each of these questions as objectively and honestly as you can.

As a manager, I (sometimes, usually, always):

	Sometimes	Usually	Always
1. Take time to listen to my employees' ideas and thoughts.	____	____	____
2. Recognize the accomplishments of employees, even if they are small.	____	____	____
3. Stay informed about what's going on in the group practice and update my employees on various things.	____	____	____
4. Clarify performance standards and communicate expectations as often as necessary.	____	____	____
5. See myself positively and act as a positive role model for my employees.	____	____	____
6. Learn about training and educational opportunities for my employees.	____	____	____
7. Provide feedback to my employees on their performance on a regular basis.	____	____	____
8. Take a genuine interest in my employees' personal and career development.	____	____	____
9. Notice when employee attitudes shift and morale is down.	____	____	____
10. Offer coaching to my employees during good times as well as difficult times for them and the group practice.	____	____	____
11. Go to employees to provide feedback and not always wait for them to come to me.	____	____	____
12. Encourage my employees to be responsible for their career and performance management.	____	____	____
13. Keep current in my industry and share new knowledge with my employees.	____	____	____
14. Commit to my own personal and professional development.	____	____	____
15. Provide consistent opportunities for performance and career development discussions with my employees.	____	____	____

Select five behaviors where you checked Sometimes or Often and where you would like to see improvement in your coaching skills. Write these down in the space provided. Make and implement an improvement plan.

1.______________________________

2.______________________________

3.______________________________

4.______________________________

5.______________________________

How to Use Coaching in Performance Management

The most important rule in coaching is that performance standards are specific, clear and mutually agreed upon. Once the standards have been established, then you have a basis for coaching. Use this step-by-step approach as a guideline for managing performance issues.

1. Identify the Need for Coaching	The first step is to determine the coaching need. Is there a performance issue with this specific employee? Does it relate to his/her career development or is it specific to a function or task? Coaching is directed at a specific need.
2. Map Your Coaching Strategy	For the second step, determine how best to approach the situation. Should your strategy include training, peer-instruction, job restructuring, reassignment, etc.? Know this before you have your coaching meeting.
3. Plan Your Coaching Meeting	The third step is to decide how much time is needed for the coaching meeting. Think about what questions you'll ask, how progress will be observed and measured.
4. Recommend Actions to the Employee	Meet with the employee and present the situation with facts or observed behavior. Ask questions that allow the employee to understand your concern. Discuss your strategy, plan and action steps.

5. Get Agreement from the Employee	Agreement is critical for performance coaching to be effective. Obtain agreement from the employee on the strategy, plan and action steps.
6. Observe the Employee 's Performance	You must personally observe the employee's performance to coach best. Otherwise, it's peer feedback, but not coaching. Determine if the strategy is effective and the action steps are being implemented.
7. Evaluate the Employee's Performance	Using the agreed-upon measures, evaluate if the employee's performance has improved.
8. Revise the Coaching Plan and/or Reward the Employee	Recognize all progress the employee has made and provide feedback as soon as possible. Make revisions to the coaching plan, if needed, and implement the plan with the employee's agreement.

Coaching Meetings

Performance coaching meetings can be easy and effective if you follow these simple rules.[11]

Planning Desired Outcomes

- The employee understands the purpose of the meeting.
- The employee recognizes your willingness to support his or her improvement.
- The employee understands the strategy, plan and action steps.
- The employee assumes responsibility for his or her part of the plan.

Planning Rules

- Know what you want to accomplish with the meeting.
- Be open and flexible to change the coaching plan if the conversation deems it appropriate.
- Review any prior performance notes or records.
- Give the employee a chance to prepare for the meeting.
- Prepare an agenda to use the meeting time effectively.

- Hold the meeting in a location where both of you will not be distracted and interrupted.
- Set aside enough time for the agenda and additional conversation.

Coaching Meeting Rules

Be direct by starting with a statement that reflects a performance issue, such as: *"I'm concerned that you're not answering the phone in a timely manner. This has created a problem for other employees and complaints from patients. I wanted to meet with you to discuss how it may be addressed."*

- Listen when the employee is talking. A good coach takes time to listen. Model appropriate listening behavior.
- Listen for both verbal and non-verbal messages. The employee may need additional support from you and have a difficult time communicating his or her needs.
- Maintain your position as the coach. Discuss your strategy, plan and action steps. Let the employee know you are interested in supporting his or her performance and will provide the necessary resources to ensure success.
- Be clear about the actions the employee must take to improve his or her performance. Provide options to the strategy or action plan, if needed.
- End the meeting with a clear understanding of the next steps, how he or she will be measured, and when the next meeting will be held.

Coaching is a critical skill for managers in building effective and motivated employees. The technique used can either be effective or ineffective in influencing performance improvement.[12] It can be used to correct inadequate performance and to reinforce and further improve appropriate performance.

Performance Mentoring

Another technique to boost employee performance is mentoring. Ambitious employees are looking for mentors who can help them navigate their career ladders and provide valuable insights within the industry. Mentors may be another manager, an executive or someone who the protégé admires for their accomplishments.

Many managers see mentoring new hires as a way to foster successful behavior and to make a direct impact on individual performance. Some employees may consider mentoring a reward as valuable as a promotion or raise. Having a mentor allows them to "remove" a few of the rungs in their career ladder and provides a path for both performance and career development.

Any practice can use mentoring as part of its performance management strategy. Here's an example of how one manager developed a mentoring relationship with a potential "star" in his organization:

Steve, the purchasing director of a mid-size HMO, hired Amanda six months ago as his administrative assistant. He noticed that Amanda was an extremely organized employee with strong decision-making skills who, with the proper training, could be groomed to be assistant purchasing director. Steve met with Amanda to discuss the possibility of her being responsible for a couple of projects that he needed to have done. He offered to help her if she encountered any difficulties.

Steve also identified a number of skills that Amanda would need to develop as part of her career path and not just for these particular projects. These included how to do cost and price analysis, how to negotiate contract terms, and how to look for red flags in supplier agreements. Amanda was excited and very interested in accepting more responsibilities and learning new skills to enhance her long-term opportunities.

They agreed to meet every two weeks in Steve's office at lunchtime—he brought in sandwiches—to discuss the status of the projects. Amanda would provide an update on the projects and share any challenges she encountered, and Steve would provide feedback and ideas for overcoming the challenges.

Steve never promised Amanda a promotion or a raise. The word "mentor" was never used, however, this was a mentoring relationship. It may be very similar to ones you may already have participated in and not considered as mentoring.

The Difference between Mentoring and Coaching

Mentoring is often confused with coaching because one of the functions of a mentor is to coach the protégé. But mentoring means taking on a higher level of responsibility. The mentor does much more than just coach the employee to do his or her job well. The primary focus of mentoring is for the mentor to share his or her experiences or wisdom and political savvy to enable the potential "star" performer to take on responsibilities beyond his or her job description.

As a manager, you should coach all employees. Mentoring is intended for your potential "star" performers who have the passion and capability for career advancement. Consider mentoring as a form of "leap-frogging" where employees have a chance to progress in their career development at a different pace than others.

The Four Roles of Mentors

1. Be a role model.
2. Coach protégés.
3. Act as the broker.
4. Be the advocate.

As a mentor, your four most important roles are:

1. **Be a role model** – You model behavior that reflects the core values of the practice. Your protégés are more likely to practice the same behaviors you model. As a manager or supervisor, you strive to meet the organizational goals and your protégés want to achieve the same goals.

2. **Coach protégés** – Your role is to clarify the practice's culture, vision and political structure so your protégés learn best practices from your experiences. This way they'll avoid some of the performance traps other employees have fallen into. You also are supportive of any ideas your protégés may have in improving workflow or ideas to save the practice expenses. You act as the "sounding board" for the protégés, acknowledging their strengths and also helping them to see their shortcomings.

3. **Act as the broker** – Your protégés don't have as many contacts as you in the organization or in the industry. By listening to their career goals, you can talk to those who can provide additional resources to support the protégés' long-term career goals. You act as counsel to them and provide a path for their professional growth.

4. **Be the advocate** – Mentors act as cheerleaders for their protégés and give them a chance to show others their capabilities. You assign them projects and give them a chance to grow professionally by actually working on important tasks for the practice. In one way, you treat them as college interns who are eager to learn the industry. In this case, protégés are ready to learn and stay with the practice to develop their skills.

Characteristics of Excellent Protégés

- Track record
- Self-initiative
- Loyal
- Desire to achieve
- Enjoys challenges
- Responsible for career growth
- Values feedback
- Identifies performance challenges and sets goals

Characteristics of Excellent Mentors

- Strong interpersonal skills
- Strong contacts in the organization
- Recognizes others accomplishments
- Supervisory skills
- Knowledgeable
- Accepts risks of mentoring
- Willing to help

The Characteristics of Excellent Mentors and Protégés

Protégés

There are certain characteristics to look for in selecting employees who are good candidates for mentoring relationships. Although protégés may be multifaceted individuals, these are characteristics they have in common:

- A strong track record for performing well (regardless of the position held currently or previously)
- Demonstrated self-initiative
- Loyal to the practice and its values
- A desire to achieve results
- Enjoys challenges and is willing to accept greater responsibility
- Accepts responsibility for career growth and development
- Values feedback—both positive and constructive
- Identifies performance challenges and sets goals to overcome them

Mentors

What makes a good mentor? In the example provided, Steve had not considered himself a "mentor" and yet he possessed key traits that have been identified in excellent mentors:

- Strong interpersonal skills (e.g., listening, communication, use of questions, supportive nonverbal behavior)
- Strong contacts in the organization and influence within the practice
- Recognizes others' accomplishments at all levels

- Excellent supervisory skills (e.g., gives consistent feedback, coaches for performance, delegates effectively, provides resources needed)
- Knowledgeable in field of practice and shares knowledge
- Accepts the risks of mentoring (e.g., trusts others' capabilities and is willing to take responsibility for others' actions)
- Willing to be available and help someone else advance in the organization (e.g., committing to time and resources, sharing knowledge, not being threatened by others' success)[13]

Deciding who to mentor

There are many employees who would benefit from mentoring. Consider these opportunities for performance mentoring for your practice:

❑ Talented but plateaued employees who could use stronger interpersonal skills.
❑ Good individual performers who should learn more effective teambuilding skills.
❑ Top team member with good technical capabilities who could improve the group's productivity if her or she learned additional software techniques.
❑ Newly hired talent who could use a better understanding of the practice's core values or strategic goals.
❑ Talented, longer-term staff members who have good ideas for the practice and would benefit from critical resources to get these ideas implemented.

Implementing Performance Mentoring

Incorporating mentoring into your performance management process isn't too difficult. Use this list to determine how your practice can implement performance mentoring:

✔ Determine possible protégé candidates and their developmental needs.
✔ Determine possible mentors and their skills, abilities and knowledge.
✔ Match the needs of protégés with the mentors who would be best suited for a mentoring relationship.

Eight Tips for Implementing Mentoring in Your Practice

1. Start with a pilot group.
2. Initiate mentoring orientations.
3. Plan for a formal mentoring program.
4. Link mentoring groups to practice goals.
5. Don't do the program by yourself.
6. Use best practices and proven resources.
7. Create a structure for mentor-protégé relationships
8. Evaluate the program.

✔ Resources that are available for mentoring relationships (e.g., training, time, meal allocation).

Once you have completed this list and decided that mentoring should be a component of your practice's performance management process, consider these implementation tips:

1. Start with a pilot group. Consider mentors and protégés who are likely to do well in a pilot setting. Good targets include new hires and budding managers.
2. Initiate mentoring orientations. Offer orientations that explain the roles of mentors and protégés, provide self-study materials and articles on mentoring, and observe managers' and employees' interest in mentoring.
3. Plan for a formal mentoring program. Organizations that have implemented performance mentoring successfully allowed for six months to plan the program and to get "buy in" from managers and employees.
4. Link mentoring goals to practice goals. Mentoring programs that aren't linked to practice or organizational goals are not taken seriously and generally fail.
5. Don't do the program by yourself. Create a task force that is interested in mentoring and its benefits. Give everyone a role and a set of tasks to implement and manage the program.
6. Use best practices and proven resources. There's no use in reinventing the wheel. Great materials for designing programs and for training mentors and protégés already exist. Look within your local library or bookstore for books like:

   - *The Mentoring Guide: Facilitating Effective Learning Relationships,* Zachary, 2000
   - *Making Mentoring Happen: A Simple and Effective Guide to Implementing a Successful Mentoring Program,* Lacey, 2000
   - *Beyond the Myths and Magic of Mentoring: How to Facilitate an Effective Mentoring Process,* Murray, 2001

   You can also check out some great mentoring websites like www.mentoringgroup.com, www.workplacetoolbox.com, or www.mentoringsolutions.com for best practice ideas, resources and consultants.

7. Create structure for mentor-protégé relationships. Have an application process, clear roles for mentors and protégés, forms to use throughout the relationship, training, materials, scheduled activities, etc. Leaving mentors and protégés to figure things out on their own will cause the initiative to fail. Start with structure and once seasoned mentors understand the process, the structure can loosen up. It's too hard to instill structure when the process started off informally. Online resources like www.workplace-toolbox.com provide forms to use in mentoring programs. They provide free downloads as well as mentoring kits with forms included on disk. (See the example of a Mentoring Progress Review in Figure 4-2.)[14]
8. Evaluate the program regularly. Checking to see how the program is working for both mentors and protégés will allow you to make needed changes. Don't wait until a whole year has passed before evaluating the program. Collect more than "feel good" data that say the program is good. Before you begin, consider getting baseline information about protégé competencies, knowledge and satisfaction with the practice, etc. Then ask protégés to measure the changes in each area as a result of performance mentoring. Review forms similar to the one used in Figure 4-2 are a great way to collect information about the mentoring relationships.

Several organizations have seen positive results from designing and implementing mentoring programs. New hires at a mid-size bank that participated in a mentoring program reduced their learning time by 25 percent compared to earlier groups. A year-long mentoring program at a manufacturing organization found that over 85 percent of the participants rated the program as "very good" or "excellent overall." Just as many protégés indicated that the program helped them achieve personal development and career enrichment goals.[15]

Figure 4-2
Progress Review for Mentors

How often do you and your protégé meet? ______________________

Indicate how and where you usually meet: (check all that apply)

___ In the protégé's office
___ In your office
___ Over breakfast/lunch
___ On the phone
___ Via email
___ While performing/observing specific job-related functions
___ Other (please specify)____________________________________

____

To date, what has been the most valuable part of mentoring for you?

____

____

Do you feel that your protégé is committed to this mentoring relationship?
____

____

Has your protégé exceeded or met your initial expectations? If not, please explain.____

____

What has been the best aspect of this mentoring partnership?_______

____

What improvements would you would recommend to enhance the mentoring program?____

____

Please add any additional insights or comments:__________________

____

____

This completed review form is placed in the protégé's personnel file for later reference. [16]

Summary

Performance mentoring initiatives and programs take time and effort to be effective. Take the time and resources to do it right and it can become an integral part of your performance management process.

In this chapter, you explored several new performance management trends, including the symbiotic relationship between self-managing careers and career development, coaching for performance and performance mentoring. Implementing these initiatives as part of your performance management strategies takes time but yields improved relationships and performance in your practice.

References:

1. C.S. Hakim, *We Are All Self-Employed,* San Francisco, CA: Barrett-Koehler, 1994.
2. Gerald Sturman, Ph.D., *Coaching Careers and Performance,* Bedford, NY: Bierman House, 1999.
3. *The Medical Practice Performance Management Manual: How to Evaluate Employees,* Englewood, CO: MGMA, 1993, p. 81.
4. Gerald Sturman, Ph.D., *Managing Your Career with Power,* Bedford, NY: Bierman House, 1999.
5. Richard Nelson Bowles, *What Color's Your Parachute?* Berkeley, CA, Ten Speed Press, 2000.
6. *The Medical Practice Performance Management Manual: How to Evaluate Employees,* Englewood, CO: MGMA, 1993, p. 99.
7. David Dotlich and Peter Cairo, "Performance in Practice," ASTD Newsletter, Fall 2000.
8. Florence Stone, *Coaching, Counseling & Mentoring: How to Choose & Use the Right Technique to Boost Employee Performance,* New York, NY: AMACOM, 1999.
9. Florence Stone, *Coaching, Counseling & Mentoring: How to Choose & Use the Right Technique to Boost Employee Performance,* New York, NY: AMACOM, 1999.
10. Gerald Sturman, Ph.D., *Coaching Careers and Performance,* Bedford, NY: Bierman House, 1999.
11. Gerald Sturman, Ph.D., *Coaching Careers and Performance,* Bedford, NY: Bierman House, 1999.

12. Florence Stone, *Coaching, Counseling & Mentoring: How to Choose & Use the Right Technique to Boost Employee Performance*, New York, NY: AMACOM, 1999.
13. The Mentoring Group, www.mentoringgroup.com.
14. www.workplacetoolbox.com.
15. www.mentoringsolutions.com.
16. Modified from the *Mentoring Progress Review*, www.workplacetoolbox.com.

Implementing a Performance Management System

Chapter 5

Implementing a Performance Management System

1. Create a vision.
2. Set expectations.
3. Provide ongoing feedback.
4. Conduct evaluation.
5. Follow up.

Performance management is an essential part of any manager's job and is important to the success of medical group practices. Implementing a performance management system in the practice assures that each employee will be judged fairly and objectively and rewarded on the basis of job performance. Performance management also helps managers identify employees for promotion as well as employees with performance problems. If necessary, performance management helps document performance problems that can lead to improvement or a fair and legal termination. The bottom line is that effective utilization of a performance management system capitalizes on organizations most important asset: *their people.*

This chapter will lay the groundwork to help any medical group practice develop and implement a performance management system. It will provide details on topics such as:

- Creating a vision
- Establishing and measuring goals and standards
- Providing feedback
- Holding a successful evaluation meeting
- Following up to ensure success

Performance management should be an ongoing process in which the manager and employee continually communicate and interact. It should result in an objective, constructive evaluation of the employee's success in meeting established goals or expectations. The following diagram identifies a structured methodology for managers to use when managing employee performance.

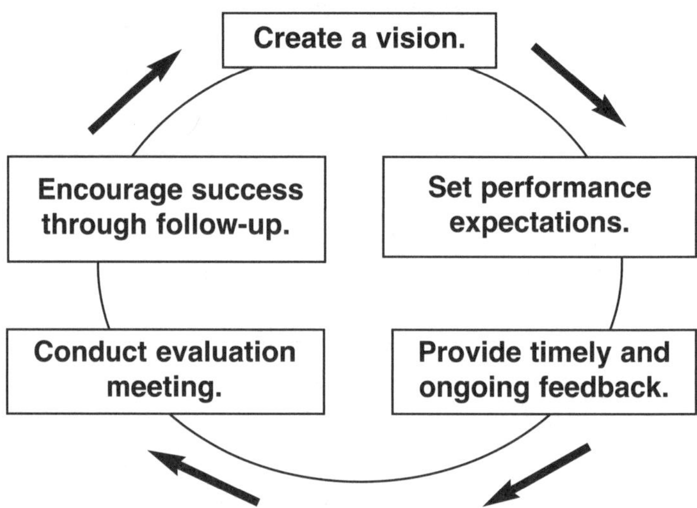

For more detailed information and guidelines on how to implement the performance management process including system procedures, supervisory training, developmental plans and process review, please refer to *The Medical Practice Performance Management Manual: How To Evaluate Employees*, Chapter 6.

How To Set Performance Expectations

Employees will perform better on the job when they clearly understand what is expected of them. Whether a new employee or an existing employee, expectations should be clearly defined and communicated to the employee. Expectations are communicated through employee job descriptions, performance standards, defined goals or preferred behaviors.[1]

Performance expectations should identify:

- Basic job responsibilities and everyday job duties as defined and outlined in the job description;

- How tasks should be performed and acceptable levels of performance for a job (i.e., performance standards); and
- Short- and long-term goals, training goals or related activities (i.e., performance objectives).

Start with the Big Picture

Strong organizations have a clear vision of where they will be in the future. Understanding that vision is vital to the success and performance of employees. Employees want to be part of a successful organization that is planning for future growth and development. Therefore, visionary individual performance expectations and how they will be measured must be clear and meaningful to employees. They need to be consistent and in alignment with the organizational goals and vision for the future.

As the manager, the first step in setting goals and expectations for your employees is to establish a vision for your department or team. This vision will identify your direction and purpose and support the overall strategic plans for the organization. Some questions to consider are:

- ❏ What are the goals of our practice in the next six months to three years? How can my team help our practice achieve those goals?
- ❏ Based on the future vision of our practice, how could my team look different five years from now?
- ❏ How is medical technology changing and what does my team need to be prepared to handle in the future?

Once you have established and agreed upon the vision for your department or team, employees will have a picture of the future and their role in it. From this point, managers and employees can develop individual goals and expectations that support achievement of reaching the strategic objectives of the department and the organization.

Communicating Performance Standards

As the manager, it is important that your expectations of how the employee should perform his or her job are clearly stated and discussed with the employee. Performance standards define to your employees what is an acceptable level of performance for their job. Standards are important because they apply measurement to how the employee performs the responsibilities outlined in his or her job description.

For example, responsibilities for an office receptionist may include:

- ❑ Return patient calls in a timely manner.
- ❑ Be friendly and informative when helping answer patient inquiries.
- ❑ Process paperwork efficiently.

You can apply standards to these job responsibilities by expressing your expectations using quantity, quality, time or cost:

- ❑ Return patient calls with 24 hours.
- ❑ Process all daily paperwork by 5 pm that day.
- ❑ Any office supply purchases over $200 must be approved by the manager.

Performance standards should always be discussed and agreed upon at the beginning of any employment relationship. However, it may also be necessary to review performance standards at any time during the performance management process if the employee is not meeting job expectations.

Criteria for Effective Goals

1. Specific
2. Measurable
3. Acceptable
4. Realistic
5. Time bound

Strategies for Effective Goal-Setting

Setting goals with employees is an essential element of effective performance management. Without goals, achievement is not easily measured. Goals are simply a clearer statement of what accomplishments must be achieved if the organization's vision is to become a reality. Goals can focus employees on the purpose of the organization; enhance chances of long-and short-term success; and motivate employees.

Goals must be:

- ❑ **Specific** - To provide enough information so employees know exactly what they should be doing to reach their goals, who is involved and why they are doing it.

Employees have a greater chance of reaching specifically defined goals rather than general goals

- ❑ **Measurable** – Defining what the end result will look like when the goal has been achieved. When progress is measurable, employees stay on track and are motivated to continue their effort in pursuit of the goal.
- ❑ **Acceptable** - Decided and agreed upon jointly by the employee and the manager. When employees decide on goals that are important to them, they have a greater interest in making them happen.
- ❑ **Realistic** – Does the employee truly believe that given the time and resources available he or she can attain the goal?
- ❑ **Time designated** – Date specified as to when the goal should be reached.

When creating goal statements, try to begin with an action verb that can be observed and measured.

Five Elements of Career Management

1. Assessment
2. Investigate
3. Match
4. Choose
5. Manage

Examples:	reduce	correct	write	increase
	produce	delegate	solve	achieve
	develop	establish	answer	control
	create	identify	assign	operate
	implement	prepare	analyze	transfer
	conduct	review	choose	process

Examples of effective goal statements:

- ❑ Reduce annual travel expenses by 10 percent by year end 2002.
- ❑ Develop a new patient filing system by December 15, 2002.
- ❑ Design and distribute a patient satisfaction survey by March 31, 2002.

Setting Goals Exercise

Develop two goal statements for you or your team. Define how they meet the criteria for effective goals and how they tie to organizational objectives.

Goal Statement #1:

How is this goal:

Specific:

Measurable:

Acceptable:

Realistic:

Time Bound:

How does this goal support organizational objectives?

Goal Statement #2:

How is this goal:

Specific:

Measurable:

Acceptable:

Realistic:

Time Bound:

How does this goal support organizational objectives?

Why Goal-Setting Fails

1. Goals are unrealistic.
2. Goals are not clearly defined.
3. Goals are sporadic.
4. Goals are not prioritized.

Why Goal Setting Fails

Goal setting can go wrong for a number of reasons:[2]

- ❑ Goals are unrealistic for the individual. If the employee feels that the goal is unreachable, the employee will not be motivated to achieve it. Conversely, if the goal is too simple, the employee may feel it's a waste of time and possibly disrespectful of his or her abilities.
- ❑ Goals are not clearly defined and therefore cannot be measured. Progress toward a goal that has not been properly defined is difficult to ascertain. Consequently, employee self-confidence in achieving the goal will be minimal.
- ❑ Goal setting is sporadic and disorganized. Goals are set to "put out fires" and achievement of goals will not be measured and feedback will not occur properly. If this happens, then the major benefits of goal setting are lost.
- ❑ Goals are not prioritized. The employee can feel overwhelmed when too many goals are not prioritized and can lose the momentum to continue toward achievement of any goals.

Remember that when goal setting fails, the possibilities of the organization and/or team meeting its goals diminishes, and employee morale and motivation drops. By avoiding these problems and setting goals effectively, you can achieve and maintain strong forward momentum toward reaching your objectives and realizing your vision.

How to Use Performance Measures With Employees

What Is Performance Measurement?

Performance measurement is a quantitative way to let a manager or organization know important information about performance. Performance measurement enables management to see the difference between "what was expected" and "what actually occurred." Managers use this tool to gather data so they can understand, manage and improve the performance in their department or team. Performance measurement provides managers with the information necessary to make intelligent decisions about what to do next.

Performance measures can let management know:

- how well employees are doing;
- if employees are achieving stated goals;
- if employees are meeting performance standards;
- if patients are satisfied; and
- if and where improvements are necessary.

Measuring Performance

1. Effectiveness
2. Efficiency
3. Quality
4. Timeliness
5. Productivity
6. Safety

Performance Measurement Categories

Most performance measures can be grouped into one of these six general categories:[3]

1. Effectiveness: Are employees doing the right things?

2. Efficiency: Are employees doing things right?

3. Quality: Is the service being provided meeting customer requirements and expectations?

4. Timeliness: Was the work done correctly and on time?

5. Productivity: What was the value added in relation to the amount of labor and capital consumed?

6. Safety: Is the working environment safe?

How To Develop Performance Measures

When defining performance measures make sure they:

- ✔ focus on what you expect to happen and what the results will look like when the goal is achieved;
- ✔ provide useful information about progress toward objectives and goals;
- ✔ are reliable and accurate; and
- ✔ are not too difficult to implement.

Performance measures can range from simple observations of employee performance to complex statistical reports and analysis. It is up to the supervisor to decide what information on performance is needed and the best way to gather that information through utilization of a performance measurement tool.

When developing performance measures:

1. Decide on what needs to be measured.
2. Define the measure, how it is calculated, what it shows and why it is important information.
3. Implement internal controls to assure that information is properly collected and reported.
4. Retain documentation that supports the performance measure reported.

How To Enhance Employee Performance Through Feedback

Observing employee performance and providing timely feedback about performance should be a routine part of the performance management process. Feedback should be based on observed and/or verifiable work-related behaviors, actions, statements and results. Ongoing feedback throughout the evaluation period reinforces desired behaviors and improves employee performance when needed.[4]

As discussed in *The Medical Practice Performance Management Manual: How To Evaluate Employees*, Chapter 7, feedback is a tool that can be used to measure progress by regularly informing employees on how they are doing in relation to their performance expectations and goals. This important information can help employees be more effective.

It has been proven that feedback is most effective when given as soon as possible after an action occurs. An employee who is not meeting expectations should be given feedback prior to the formal performance evaluation meeting, since unanticipated information can create conflict and hard feelings. Keep in mind, **there should never be any surprises at the evaluation meeting**. By keeping the lines of communication open between employees and management a climate of mutual understanding is established where job satisfaction and increased productivity will flourish.

As illustrated in Figure 5.1, feedback has to be part of two-way communication to make sure information is clearly understood by both the sender and the receiver.

Figure 5.1
Feedback loop

True two-way communication involves a feedback loop; i.e., supervisor and employee send messages back and forth to ensure each "hears" and understands the other.

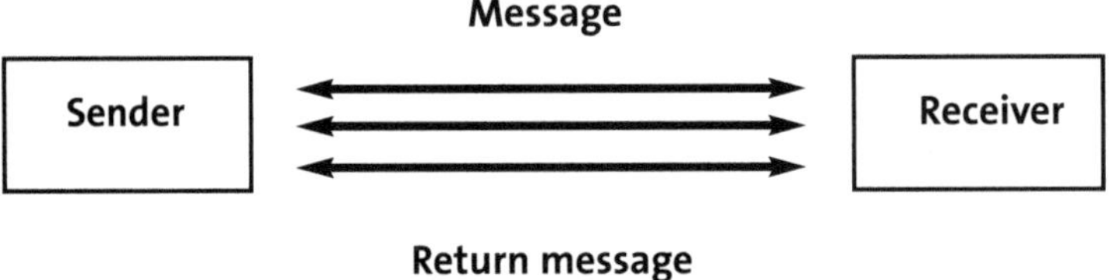

Based on classic communication model.

Source: *The Medical Practice Performance Management Manual: How To Evaluate Employees,* page 134.

Types of Feedback

- ❑ Behavioral
- ❑ Positive
- ❑ Corrective

Types of Feedback

When observing employee performance, the manager has the opportunity to give effective feedback on work-related behaviors and activities.[5] These behaviors can be positive or corrective based on if they are contributing to or hindering the progress toward achievement of employee goals. Feedback based on observed performance is much more likely to influence employee behavior than feedback that cannot be supported by first-hand information. That is why management by walking around (MBWA) is so important in any organization. Effective feedback can help employees achieve success and motivate them to develop new skills, knowledge or experience. Observation techniques are explained in more detail in the book *The Medical Practice Performance Management Manual: How To Evaluate Employees,* Chapter 7.

Behavioral Feedback

When giving employees feedback on work-related behaviors, it is meant to be influential.[6] The objective is to influence the employee to continue the same successful behaviors or to eliminate any behavior causing problems. Regular and ongoing feedback for both positive and negative behaviors will establish a bond of trust and mutual respect between supervisor and employee. When employees receive feedback that is timely, frequent and specific, they are more likely to understand what is expected of them, to repeat successful performance and to improve their work when necessary.

It is imperative that behavioral feedback provides specific examples of behaviors, not an evaluation of personality or judgment about what the behavior means. Compare these statements:

- ❑ *You have a great attitude when dealing with patients.*
- ❑ *You smile when greeting the patient, refer to them by name, say please when asking for information and thank you when receiving information.*[7]

In the first example, the supervisor has evaluated a personality trait and has not offered the employee any information that is useful as feedback. In the second example, the supervisor states facts and observations about the behavior so that in the future the employee will know what exactly what is considered appropriate and positive behavior. The supervisor is recognizing behavior that should be repeated.

Exercise

1. Compare two responses.
2. Put your notes in the box.

Tips To Giving Behavioral Feedback

- ✔ Be specific.
- ✔ Be timely.
- ✔ Ask for employee input.
- ✔ Work together.
- ✔ Share the impact.
- ✔ Be supportive.

How Can You Change These Statements to Behaviors?

After reading the two responses, compare them in the box provided.

Typical Response: "You never meet our customer needs."

Recommended Response: "This week two new customers called to complain that you did not return their phone call for three days."

Typical Response: "Your performance is outstanding."

Recommended Response: "Each day you come to work on time, process and file all your paperwork by the end of each day, and ask your co-workers how you can assist them with their daily tasks."

Typical Response: "You have a bad attitude that is affecting the team."

Recommended Response: "Twice this week you stated out loud that no one except you is following procedures correctly in the office. You used a loud and discerning voice tone. Team members in the office discussed with me that your comments make them feel that they are doing a poor job at work."

When giving behavioral feedback, follow these guidelines:[8]

1. Give feedback on specific, observable or verifiable data.
2. Give feedback as close to the event at possible.
3. After describing the observed behavior, ask for employee input as to why the behavior is occurring.

Corrective Feedback

- ✔ Discuss behavior.
- ✔ Explain effect.
- ✔ Clarify expectations.
- ✔ Agree on outcomes of change.

4. Work together to overcome problems or ideas on how to improve.
5. Share the impact of the behavior on the team, department or organization.
6. Be supportive.

Positive Feedback

Positive feedback is important to encourage behavior and performance that you want to see continued. As noted in *The Medical Practice Performance Management Manual: How To Evaluate Employees,* Chapter 7, pages 127-128, experts suggest that supervisors use the 80/20 ratio, with feedback consisting of 80 percent positive reinforcement and 20 percent aimed at improvement. Always give positive feedback when employee performance:

- ✔ Shows improvement, even if it doesn't yet fully meet expectations.
- ✔ Consistently meets expectations.
- ✔ Exceeds expectations.

Corrective Feedback

The goals in giving corrective feedback are to eliminate the behavior that caused the problem and to get the employee back on track so he or she can contribute to the team's success. Using the following approach lets the employee know that you care and want to help improve performance:

- ✔ Discuss the behavior.
- ✔ Explain how the behavior is affecting the team or organization.
- ✔ Clarify what is the expected behavior.
- ✔ Agree on what the outcome of changing behavior will look like.

Many supervisors may find that giving corrective feedback is difficult because they are afraid of hurting feelings or creating conflict between the employee and supervisor. However, it is important to realize that by giving corrective feedback when needed, the supervisor is offering critical information that is providing the employee with the chance to improve.

As illustrated in Figure 5.2, supervisors can test their feedback skills by referring to this Feedback Problem Checklist.

Figure 5.2
Feedback Problem Checklist

The list of feedback problems helps supervisors check their effectiveness in giving feedback and gives them clues about skill-building needs.

Avoidance

- ✔ Avoids giving any feedback.
- ✔ Avoids giving negative feedback.
- ✔ Avoids giving positive feedback.

Comparison

- ✔ Compares one employee against another.

Criticism

- ✔ Attacks the person rather than the behavior.
- ✔ Criticizes several things at once rather than one at a time.
- ✔ Sandwiches negative comments in between positive feedback.
- ✔ Criticizes employees in front of others.

Sensitivity

- ✔ Ignores the employee's receptivity to feedback.
- ✔ Emphasizes own point of view and does not seek employee's.
- ✔ Focuses on proving the supervisor is right rather than finding the cause of the employee's behavior.
- ✔ Uses sarcasm and caustic remarks.
- ✔ Interrupts employee when he or she is responding to the feedback.
- ✔ Gives little consideration to the impact the feedback may have on the future relationship with the employee.

Timing

- ✔ Delays giving feedback until a long time after the incident.
- ✔ Gives feedback when angry, tense or tired.

Clarification

- ✔ Forgets to check to see if the employee "got the message."

Attitude

- ✔ Feels it is more important to give feedback than to receive it.
- ✔ Feels it is more important to point out mistakes than to problem-solve how to correct them.

Method

- ✔ Prefers to give feedback in writing rather than orally, face-to-face.

Source: *The Medical Practice Performance Management Manual: How To Evaluate Employees*, page 139

How to Have a Successful Performance Evaluation Meeting

A performance evaluation is a review of individual job behaviors and performance results to determine if performance was effective. It identifies employees capable of performing, employees who require more training, and employees who do not meet performance standards. Evaluations assist in compensation and staffing decisions, as well as offer direction for future performance.

Preparation Tips

- ❑ Gather information.
- ❑ Compare information with expectations and goals.
- ❑ Notify employee of evaluation.
- ❑ Set up meeting.
- ❑ Determine message.
- ❑ Anticipate reaction.
- ❑ Complete management evaluation.
- ❑ Establish outline.

Preparation

Communicating expectations, giving day-to-day feedback, documenting actual performance and preparing for the performance evaluation will help to make for a successful performance evaluation meeting. The key to a well-prepared, effective evaluation is having objective, job-specific data that support the ratings given on the evaluation form. Information to help supervisors prepare and plan for the performance evaluation is outlined in the following checklists. [9]

Planning Performance Evaluation Meeting Checklist

- ✓ Gather and review all applicable performance data and information. This information could include the job description, agreed-upon performance standards, performance diaries, rewards or recognition, and customer kudos or complaints.
- ✓ Compare information to expectations and goals that have been set.
- ✓ Notify employee in advance to complete self-evaluation. The self-evaluation gives the employees an opportunity to assess their own performance throughout the review period.
- ✓ Schedule evaluation meeting. The evaluation meeting should take place in a neutral setting. This may be in a conference room, restaurant over lunch, or an empty office.
- ✓ Determine what your message to the employee will be. What do you want the employee thinking, feeling and doing when he or she leaves the meeting?

- ✓ Anticipate employee reaction. Is the employee going to be surprised? If so, then there probably was not enough feedback and communication between the employee and manager throughout the year.
- ✓ Complete the management evaluation review.
- ✓ Establish outline for meeting. What is the length of time for the evaluation meeting? (Most evaluation meetings are no more than 45 minutes to 1 hour.) Leave time for discussion of the management assessment, employee input, and future goals and objectives.

Preparing For Employee Evaluation

By answering the following questions, a manager can establish a clear picture of employee performance and any obstacles that may have hindered success or progress during the evaluation period. Taking these answers into account can lead to a fair and honest performance evaluation.

Have you done your job as the manager? Ask yourself the following:

- Have you worked together with your employee to set goals for the year?
- Were these goals acceptable and achievable by the employee?
- Are you aware of any problems that prevented the employee from meeting goals?
- Have you established measures to determine if the goals have been reached?
- Have you been supportive in helping employee meet goals?
- Have you provided the employee with regular and ongoing feedback on their performance?
- Has your employee felt comfortable enough to regularly come to you with questions or raise concerns?
- Have you been available and accessible for your employees?
- Has your own performance served as a role model for your employee?
- Have you maintained documentation on employee performance throughout the year that you can reference?
- Are you prepared to give specific examples of any behavioral issues or performance problems that will be discussed?
- Have you considered and developed an improvement plan with suggestions for problem areas?

Has the employee done his or her job? Ask yourself the following:

- Does the employee have the knowledge, skills and abilities necessary to do the job?
- Could the employee be doing a better a job? How?
- Does the employee need additional training?
- Are the expectations for the job being met?
- What are the employee's strong areas?
- What are the areas where the employee could improve?
- What contributions is the employee making to the team or the practice?
- What contributions should the employee be making to the team or practice?

The Seven-Step Evaluation Discussion

Step 1:
Control the environment.

Step 2:
State the purpose.

Step 3:
Ask for employee's assessment.

Step 4:
Present your assessment.

Step 5:
Ask for employee's reaction.

Step 6:
Set specific goals.

Step 7:
Close the discussion.

Holding a Successful Evaluation Meeting

A successful evaluation meeting depends greatly on your skill as a discussion leader.[9] An effective discussion leader encourages two-way discussions and works to keep the channels of communication open. When the meeting is over, both parties should have a better understanding of each other and how their job performance is related. Remember that the best approach during this part of the process is to act as a coach to your employee.

How to Hold a Successful Evaluation Meeting

1. Control the environment:
   a. The meeting should be kept confidential.
   b. Allow ample time for meeting.
   c. Minimize all interruptions.
   d. Conduct the meeting as close to the review date as possible (within one week).
   e. Put the employee at ease by opening with questions about something other than work to let the employee know you care about him or her as an individual.
2. State the purpose of the evaluation meeting.
3. Ask for employee's assessment of own performance:
   a. Ask for clarification on any information in self-evaluation.
   b. Present management assessment of employee performance.

   c. Build on employee's strengths focusing on areas where the employee has excelled or shown improvement.
   d. Be candid and kind, discussing specific examples of both positive and negative performance or behavioral issues.
   e. Discuss the role and responsibilities of the employee and how his or her performance impacts the department and the practice as a whole.
   f. Show confidence in the employee's ability to improve in problem areas and support to continue to show success in positive performance areas.
5. Ask for the employee's reaction:
   a. Allow employee to voice opinions.
   b. Listen to employee's concerns.
   c. Answer questions.
   d. Ask questions for clarification if needed.
6. Set goals for upcoming evaluation period:
   a. Work together with employee.
   b. Agree on goals.
7. Close evaluation meeting:
   a. End on a positive note.

Purpose of Follow-up

- ✔ To Change Goals or Standards
- ✔ To Review Action Plans
- ✔ To Discuss Progress
- ✔ To Schedule Training
- ✔ To Give Positive Feedback

The Importance of Follow-Up

Follow-up after the performance appraisal meeting or at any time during the review period may be appropriate. Effective managers don't wait for their employees to come to them - they go to their employees. Managers who frequently interact and communicate with their employees tend to have fewer employee performance problems.

Frequent follow-up with your employees tells them you think they are important. The way you communicate with your employees demonstrates how much you care about them as people – not just as employees. Sometimes you have to go out of your way to interact with your employees, but they always will notice how much effort you put forth to communicate with them.

Purposes of follow-up after a performance evaluation could include the following:

- ❑ To reset or change standards or objectives;
- ❑ To review action plan to reach goals;
- ❑ To plan or discuss progress toward improved performance;
- ❑ To schedule training; and
- ❑ To give employee positive feedback on progress.

Summary

In summary, supervisors can make the difference in employee attitude and performance. Establishing standards and goals, providing appropriate and timely feedback and making sure to follow up throughout the performance period are critical components necessary for superior performance. It is the job of the supervisor to continually try to develop employees to their full potential using all of the components of the performance management process.

References:

1. *Performance Appraisal Design,* Presented by Mountain States Employers Council, Inc., Denver, CO: MSEC, 1998.
2. On-line: http://madgopes.com/goalsfailure.html
3. On-line: Oakridge Associated Universities http://www.orau.gov/pbm/Default.htmThe Medical Practice
4. *The Medical Practice Performance Management Manual: How to Evaluate Employees,* Englewood, CO: MGMA, 1993.
5. On-line: University of California, San Diego http://blink-prod.ucsd.edu/Blink/External/Topics/How_To/1,1260,737,00.html
6. On-line: University of California, San Diego http://wwwhr.ucsd.edu/~staffeducation/guide/obsfdbk.html#Behavioral
7. *Performance Appraisal Design,* Presented by Mountain States Employers Council, Inc., Denver, CO: MSEC, 1998.
8. On-line: University of California, San Diego http://www-hr.ucsd.edu/~staffeducation/guide/obsfdbk.html#Behavioral
9. *The Performance Appraisal.* Business & Legal Reports, Inc. 1997.

Compensation Strategies

Chapter 6

"At a time of economic slowdowns and uncertainty, a compensation concept such as pay for performance is particularly tempting and increasingly popular...It's an understandable trend at a time when revenues slump, stock options shrivel, and across-the-board raises just isn't feasible for many organizations."—Janet Wiscombe, 2001 [1]

Compensation strategies should be part of your performance management system to recognize and reward employees for meeting performance standards. This chapter will provide an overview of various performance pay plans and how they can be used to align individual and team performance to group practice goals.

Compensation and its Impact on Performance

In today's competitive health care marketplace, both medical group practices and employees are aware of the important role reward and recognition strategies play in attracting and retaining talent. Using compensation as part of your performance management strategies not only offers an incentive for employees to perform, it can also enhance your performance management system.

Compensation strategies, when implemented effectively, can enhance your performance management system by:

- ✓ Focusing employees' attention on performance standards.
- ✓ Solving motivational and performance problems by providing incentives for excellent performance.
- ✓ Recognizing and rewarding positive achievements.
- ✓ Minimizing poor performance by developing a plan to positively change behavior.
- ✓ Maximizing compensation dollars by linking performance to pay.
- ✓ Attracting and retaining outstanding employees who are more likely to stay with the organization and be positive role models.

Strategically Designed Pay

Compensation is a significant investment for all group practices. Besides providing a base salary for your employees, pay plans are powerful tools that also help practices recognize and reward employees for their performance that contributes to desired business results. Therefore, strategically designed pay systems link employee contributions to results.

What are your group practice's compensation strategies and how they are aligned with your performance management system? Rate your practice's compensation strategies by responding to the following questions and comparing your score to the scale at the end of Figure 6-1.

Figure 6-1
Rate Your Practice's Compensation Strategies

Strategic pay is an integral part of an organization's compensation strategy. To review your practice's compensation strategy, answer these questions:

1. Does the practice have a wage and salary administration process?
   - ❑ Yes
   - ❑ No
2. Is this plan communicated to all employees?
   - ❑ Yes
   - ❑ No
3. Does the practice survey the local community and industry compensation rates?
   - ❑ Yes
   - ❑ No
4. Does the practice adjust compensation in line with strategic goals?
   - ❑ Yes
   - ❑ No
5. Does the practice use performance-based pay plans?
   - ❑ Yes
   - ❑ No
6. Does it offer:
   - ❑ Variable pay
   - ❑ Team incentives or bonuses
   - ❑ Competency-based pay
   - ❑ Gainsharing/results sharing
   - ❑ Skill-based pay
   - ❑ Provider performance pay
7. Do wages reflect differences in ability, responsibility, experience, effort and working conditions?
   - ❑ Yes
   - ❑ No
8. Does the practice reward performance based on specific expectations?
   - ❑ Yes
   - ❑ No
9. Does the practice use pay strategies to retain star performers?
   - ❑ Yes
   - ❑ No
10. Does your practice review its compensation plan regularly?
    - ❑ Yes
    - ❑ No

If you answered, "yes" to most questions, your practice has a strong foundation for its compensation plan.[2]

Elements of a Total Pay System

- Base-Pay
- Performance-Based Variable Pay
- Long-term Incentive Compensation
- Benefits
- Perks & Non-Cash Rewards
- Intrinsic Rewards

To attract and retain the best possible employees, practices should have a compensation system that allows them to pay for good talent and reward for performance. A compensation system encompasses total pay that includes salaries, benefits, bonuses, incentive programs and non-cash awards.

An effective total compensation system should have a combination of elements designed to support the practice's compensation philosophy and motivate and reward performance aligned with its goals and objectives. A compensation philosophy defines the practice's market position for competitive pay levels and its commitment to motivate and reward employee contribution and performance. For example, one small clinic's philosophy is "keeping critical talent happy and motivated while improving performance and providing quality patient care."

Once the compensation philosophy has been established, the practice can decide how to use strategic pay elements as part of a total pay program given the practice's objectives, operating environment and culture. The different elements of strategic pay are now described. Consider what elements your practice already has in place and which ones would be of value to incorporate as part of your compensation strategy.

Base Pay—Salary for standard job duties, skills and results. Base pay is designed to reflect competitive rates for comparable jobs within the practice's marketplace. Group practices should align their base pay programs with competitive rates in their geographic area.

Several consulting organizations conduct periodic surveys to assess current health care compensation plans, such as Boston-based Olney Associates (www.olneyassociates.com) and Price Waterhouse Coopers in New York (www.pwchealth.com). The Hay Group conducted a total compensation study in 1997 for Hospital & Health Networks Magazine.[3] The Medical Group Management Association (MGMA) also conducts compensation studies.

Performance-Based Variable Pay— Designed to reward employees for achieving specific practice and/or individual performance goals. This type of performance pay plan typically pays out in cash. Performance may be measured on an annual basis although practices can measure and reward on a monthly, quarterly or semi-annual basis. Award amounts vary from period to period depending on the practice and/or individual performance.

Types of variable pay plans include:

- Skill pay (or pay-for-knowledge, is a compensation system that bases salaries and wage rates on the repertoire of skills an employee demonstrates or applies to his/her job—such as medical claims processing or data entry).
- Incentive pay/bonus plans (form of variable compensations designed to reward accomplishments of specified performance results—such as maintaining an average of seeing 2.5 patients/hour for a given period of time).
- Gainsharing/results sharing (sharing productivity gains with employees that result in better use of labor, capital, materials and energy—such as reducing the amount of downtime or non-billable activity).

Long-term Incentive Compensation—Designed to reward long-term practice performance usually offered as stocks or stock options. Individual job level and performance may impact the eligibility of employee participation, as this incentive is generally offered to senior levels in an organization or for key talent and critical hires. This is often used as a retention tool and to promote long-term employment with the practice.

Benefits—Broad range of offerings including health and dental insurance, vacation, leave policies and retirement and savings plans. Designed to care for the health and welfare needs of employees, benefits send a strong message about the practice's culture and values.[4]

You can review the mandatory benefits that your group practice must offer its employees at the U.S. Department of Labor's web site at www.dol.gov. For information on new benefits and creative offerings, check out Old Saybrook, CT-based Benefits Next. Another useful web site, is at www.benefitsnext.com. Creative new benefits directed at retaining nurses can be explored at www.workforce.com.[5] Best practices in benefits offered by other health care organizations can be found in collective research from MGMA, including a 1999 study of 312 group practices and their benefit plans.

Perks and Non-Cash Rewards—Used to recognize exceptional performance, contribution and commitment to the practice's culture and values. Exceptional performance means something different to each group practice. For practices focused on retaining nurses, commitment rewards are used to lower turnover ratios.[6] Other practices reward employees who perform consistently high on performance evaluations using a forced-rating system. Rewards vary from additional time off, educational assistance, monthly outings, and tickets to events, dinners, public recognition, etc.

Intrinsic Rewards—Used to communicate and align employee behavior with practice priorities and values to achieve desired results. These rewards play an important role in engaging employees' skills and abilities and are critical in retaining key talent.

Types of intrinsic rewards:

- Performance feedback (provided during performance reviews, coaching sessions, or as result of observing behavior and performance on the job);
- Development opportunities (specialized training, ongoing skills and certifications); and
- Work environment and culture (an environment that allows employees to perform, stay motivated and achieve job satisfaction).

This chapter focuses primarily on performance-based variable pay. Chapter 7 describes rewards and recognition strategies that may be used as part of your practice's total pay program.

Types of Performance-Based Variable Pay

- Variable Pay
- Team Incentives or Bonuses
- Competency-Based Pay
- Gainsharing/Results Sharing
- Skill-Based Pay
- Provider Performance Pay

Performance-Based Variable Pay

In recent years, the use of various performance pay plans has increased among organizations as a more effective way to recognize and reward employee performance. Performance pay plans help to align an organization's resources and business objectives. Whether short-term or long-term, these pay plans provide an opportunity to create a common focus for employees and sustain a culture in which employees are recognized for their contributions and successes.

There are several different performance pay plan models for organizations to choose from. Your practice should determine the overall objectives it wants to achieve and select the pay plans accordingly. As with base-pay levels, assessing market trends in your area will help you identify the most popular and effective plans.[7] Check with MGMA for market trends and performance pay plans currently used with similar health care organizations. The following list provides a description of popular performance pay models used in many organizations. In this chapter, we'll explore a few of them in depth.

Variable Pay—Commonly paid out as cash awards on an annual, semi-annual or quarterly basis. Awards are generally determined based on a combination of individual performance and organization performance against pre-established goals.

Team Incentives or Bonuses—Used to reward project or team members based on the achievement of specific team goals. Payouts may be offered when project milestones have been met or the successful completion of specified performance periods, such as months or quarters. This performance pay plan is most effective when the whole team participates and specific roles and expected contributions are well defined. The award is generally the same for all team members and is usually based on either a flat dollar amount or a percentage of one's pay.

Competency-Based Pay—Pay based on the demonstration of competencies, skills and behaviors specifically identified by the practice as critical to achieve its goals. This performance pay plan is generally used to develop a more skilled workforce and complements a training and development plan.

Gainsharing/Results Sharing—Typically cash awards based on meeting specific performance objectives that are either operational and/or financial in nature. Employees "share" in the gain/result caused by their cumulative contribution—meaning it requires all employees to participate to win. This performance pay plan is generally used to increase productivity, streamline operations, or to meet cost-savings initiatives.

Skill-Based Pay—Pay based on acquiring and applying specific skills critical to the organization's operations. Although this pay plan started in manufacturing environments, it is now spreading to professional, technical, service and administrative jobs. This performance pay plan is targeted to improve the technical capabilities of employees and to encourage cross-functional training.

Provider Performance Pay—Physicians and other patient providers' pay are based on base salary, plus incentives for productivity, patient satisfaction, quality, cost savings or utilization measures.[8] Quality measures are becoming more and more an integral part of pay packages because they have a long-term effect on a practice's reputation and patient referrals. Many practices pay 5-10 percent of total compensation based on quality measures such as patient satisfaction and quality of care. These measures can also make practices better places to work because they attract employees with similar values. [9]

For additional information on physician pay plans, review articles in the *Physician Compensation Report* (access online at www.ManagedCareNewsWeb.com) or look into physician compensation education programs offered by MGMA. Your practice may also consider working with compensation consultants in your market area.

Variable Pay Plans

A survey by Hewitt Associates conducted in 2000 found that eight out of ten organizations surveyed have some type of variable pay plan, up from five out of ten in 1990. Because across-the-board raises aren't feasible for many organizations, variable pay plans are more tempting and increasingly popular. [10]

Variable Pay Benefits

This is one of the most innovative ways of bringing wages and salaries in line with practice performance. Variable pay plans are based on rewarding employees who meet performance standards and providing incentives for others to emulate. Variable pay rewards the individual worker, or in some cases, a team for its efforts. Additional benefits for practices include:

- Salaries may remain constant and not have to increase each year.
- Variable pay is re-earned each period (i.e., monthly, quarterly, annually).
- Individuals who meet performance standards consistently receive more pay than others in the same position.
- Variable pay plans with a team component encourage individual workers to strive to work together effectively. [11]

How to Structure a Variable Pay Plan

Variable pay is anchored to a measurement of performance, whether it's how many patients are seen on a monthly basis to how well a manager fosters teamwork. Performance measures may be financial (i.e., dollar amount of claims followed, revenues, expenses) and/or non-financial (i.e., maintaining attendance, meeting project deadlines, meeting customer expectations). Most organizations offering a variable pay plan use a best to worst forced-ranking system to identify and reward strong performers and encourage everyone else to work harder and smarter.

If your practice prefers to use variable pay to reward individual performance, a performance evaluation process encompassing an evaluation method such as BARS (similar to the model presented in MGMA's *Medical Practice Performance Management Manual: How to Evaluate Employees*) can be used to rate employee performance. Employees are evaluated against pre-determined goals and objectives. Using the rating scale, managers and supervisors determine how each employee is meeting his or her individual performance standards and reward accordingly.

Model 1

For example, one health plan organization uses a BARS evaluation method to rate employee performance on a scale of 1–5, with 5 being the highest, for each performance standard. Its variable pay plan then rewards employees by giving them a percentage of their quarterly salary based on their overall average ratings as follows:

- ❑ 5 percent for ratings of 4.5 or higher
- ❑ 4 percent for ratings between 3.5 and 4.4

- 3 percent for ratings between 2.5 and 3.4
- 0 percent for ratings 2.4 or less

In other organizations, variable pay plans are structured to foster meeting individual, team and practice goals. Besides receiving base pay, employees may also receive variable pay if they meet their own individual performance goals, the team meets its goals, and/or the practice achieves its organizational goals. Employees may receive bonuses for each or all goals met. (See Model 2.) This type of tiered incentive plan allows employees to succeed on three different levels of performance.

Model 2

A health care provider uses this structure of variable pay to offer employees semi-annual rewards for meeting any or all of its tiered performance goals. Employees can be rewarded on all levels and earn an additional five percent of their semi-annual salaries split as follows:

- 50 percent of the five percent if an employee meets his or her individual performance objectives.
- 40 percent of the five percent if the team meets its performance objectives.
- 10 percent of the five percent if the practice meets its performance objectives.

Using this structure, employees may be rewarded by just their own performance and have more to gain if the team and practice also achieve their goals. This encourages teamwork and is an incentive for the practice to meet its overall goals too.

Variable pay plans tie employee compensation directly to practice priorities. Because they link rewards to the achievements of specific goals and measures, variable pay plans provide flexibility to vary total pay from year to year based on the practice's strategy and results.

Flexibility allows practices to:

- Respond to changing goals and objectives;
- Create a positive partnership with employees; and
- Share success when results are achieved.

Variable pay creates a culture in which employees are rewarded for their objectives based on pre-determined objectives. It is tied closely to performance criteria. Therefore, having an effective performance management system in place is critical to the success of variable pay plans.

Five Characteristics That Predict Individual Performance

- Knowledge
- Skills
- Motives
- Traits
- Self-concepts

Competency-Based Pay Plans

Many organizations are considering or have adopted a "pay for competency" plan to reward employees for having or developing the skills, knowledge and personal characteristics and behaviors needed to perform their roles effectively. Competencies clarify performance expectations and define what knowledge and skills are necessary to do a specific job and address behaviors that have the most direct impact on job performance.[12] Excellent performers demonstrate these behaviors more consistently than average or poor performers. A competency is defined as a behavior or a set of behaviors that describe excellent performance in a particular role. Competencies differ from knowledge and skills. ***Knowledge*** is information about the specific content required in one's job—such as a surgeon's knowledge of nerves and muscles in the human body—and ***skill*** is the ability to perform a physical or mental task necessary for a position—such as a dentist's skill to fill a tooth without damaging a nerve or a psychologist's skills to provide therapeutic help.

Using a competency-based model for performance pay allows practices to "raise the bar" for performance expectations, align individual behavior with practice strategies, and lets employees understand how to achieve performance standards. This pay plan also allows practices to hire the best available people, maximize their productivity, enhance the performance appraisal process and adapt to organizational change. [13]

According to the book, *"Competence at Work,"* Spencer and Spencer state that besides knowledge and skill, three other underlying characteristics predict individual job performance. Motives, traits and self-concepts are "competencies" that differentiate superior from average performance. Knowledge and skills are important, but competencies produce success behaviors necessary for individuals and practices to succeed. Spencer and Spencer describes these three competencies as follows:

- ❑ Motives are things employees think about or want, such as achievement, that drive their behavior.
- ❑ Traits are physical characteristics and consistent responses to people or situations, such as reaction to change or customer service interactions.
- ❑ Self-concepts define an employee's attitudes, values, or self-image and may be portrayed through self-confidence or opinions. [14]

The benefits of using competency-based pay plans

Rewarding key competencies as part of your compensation strategy offers many benefits for the practice, managers and all your employees.

For the practice, the benefits include:

- Reinforcing strategy, culture and values.
- Establishing expectations for performance excellence.
- Increasing the effectiveness of training and development by linking them to specific behavior criteria.
- Providing a common understanding of the requirements of specific roles.
- Offering common, organization-wide standards for employees to move across functions and jobs.

Managers and supervisors benefit by:

- Identifying performance criteria and expectations for new hires and other employees.
- Providing more objective performance standards.
- Clarifying performance expectations to direct reports.
- Providing a foundation for dialog to discuss performance, development and career-related issues.

Employees use competency-based plans for:

- Identifying standards of performance required to be successful in their jobs.
- Supporting an objective assessment of their strengths and identifying targeted areas for professional development
- Providing the basis for more meaningful dialog with their manager or supervisor about performance, development and career-related issues.

Evaluate What Counts

First edition emphasizes performance standards

How competency is measured

Similar to variable pay plans, employees are evaluated on a regular basis using a forced-rating scale. The competency-based pay plan can evaluate the same performance measures as variable pay plans, although most organizations use competencies to rate preferred employee behavior and not financial objectives. Peers and managers/supervisors generally act as the evaluators for employee competencies. Examples of competency-based evaluations can be found in MGMA's *The Medical Practice Performance Management Manual: How to Evaluate Employees.*

Spencer and Spencer list many common competencies found in the workplace. These may form the basis for your practice's competency-based pay plan. For each position, your practice should determine the competencies an employee must perform well to meet the practice's strategy and objectives.[15]

Some competencies may be directly related for managers and supervisors, while others are competency expectations for all employees. The actual wording of competencies is determined by the practice and should be understood by all employees. Anntoinette Lucia's book, *The Art and Science of Competency Models: Pinpointing Critical Success Factors in Organizations* provides an excellent resource to develop a competency-based model for your practice.[16] You can also seek assistance from an organizational development consultant in your area by searching listings under "compensation consultants" from local directories or on the Internet.

A performance management process is comprised of steps that include planning, managing, evaluating and rewarding performance. Competency definitions are almost always used in performance management to describe employee behaviors and skills. The competency descriptions provided by Spencer and Spencer are good examples. These defined competencies allow employees to align their activities to the practice's strategies.

Gainsharing/Results Sharing Plans

Organizations generally use performance pay plans for two main reasons: (1) to manage base pay increases; and (2) to tie a portion of each employee's pay to performance. Here is how gainsharing or results sharing plans differ from other performance pay plan models:

- Gains are measured and distributions are made frequently through a predetermined formula.
- Gains are calculated in labor hours, increased productivity or decreased costs.
- Gains are based upon group, not individual performance.
- They encourage teamwork and cooperation since the whole group has to perform to earn gain payouts.
- Payouts are more frequent, usually monthly to tie performance with payments.
- Gain factors are controllable by the group members.
- They discourage competition among team members since all gains are paid out equally to everyone.

Gainsharing plans often fail because organizations determine the formula for calculating gains but don't have a structured way for all employees to be involved. Many consultants discourage gainsharing unless it requires ongoing structure to support employee participation. Effective gainsharing plans have employees involved in all aspects of its design and implementation, including identifying and solving problems, soliciting, evaluating and implementing employee suggestions and managing the group's performance. If the entire group needs to participate for everyone to be paid, members want to be involved in the whole process.[17]

In the health care industry, gainsharing has different applications. More commonly it's been used to describe a variety of compensation arrangements designed to align incentives for medical groups and physicians to provide cost-effective care and to share in cost savings through a combination of percentage payments, hourly fees or fixed fees. From the practice's perspective, gainsharing helps to lower costs—improve operational efficiencies and improve the quality of care by standardizing procedures and medical protocols.

Physicians have an opportunity to share in the gains by meeting pre-approved measures for operating margins, expense targets and satisfying quality assurance objectives. However, not all specialists can participate in such programs and tracking gains for medical organizations and physicians requires sophisticated accounting systems. Current regulations frown on paying physicians for limiting necessary medical services. [18]

Because the Office of Inspector General (OIG) and the Center for Medicine and Medicaid Services scrutinize gainsharing pay plans, practices should consult with legal counsel before implementing plans involving physicians. Although they can be designed and managed effectively, many gainsharing plans also use an independent third-party auditor to evaluate amounts earned by physicians and other health care providers.

Gainsharing plans not involving physicians or other providers of patient care can be designed and implemented effectively. *The Gainsharing Workbook* (2000) by Boyett & Boyett is an excellent source for walking through best practices for gainsharing pay plans that have been used in other industries. Just remember that group process is the key to making this type of performance pay plan effective.

Provider Performance Pay Plans

The Institute for the Future, a San Francisco not-for-profit research group, predicts that health plans and intermediaries will design reimbursement systems that provide physicians and other providers "incentives to deliver care in a manner that improves quality care, customer satisfaction, patients' tenure in the plan, and outcomes." Productivity and cost-effectiveness will also be measured because fee-for-service and capitation are not sustainable long term.

Fee-for-service payments are inflationary and capitation generates a fear of undertreatment.[19]

Keep in mind that incentive pay plans developed to motivate physicians to lower provider costs must be designed with government laws and regulations in mind. Rewards cannot be legally interpreted as kickbacks or self-referrals. Providers should not receive financial rewards for withholding services or for referring services where they have a financial interest. Your practice should check with its administrator or legal counsel to ensure that provider performance pay plans comply with current laws and regulations that govern the health care industry.

Regardless of which compensation strategy your practice selects, use the following criteria to gauge its effectiveness:

- The strategy supports the business goals of the practice.
- The strategy provides a clear link between practice goals and individual performance criteria.
- Performance expectations are communicated to all employees.
- The strategy operates without bias to individuals and has channels for questions and complaints.
- Compensation policies are established and adhered.

Summary

In this chapter, you learned about various compensation strategies to use with your performance management system. Most of the emphasis was on performance pay plans, particularly variable pay, competency-based pay and gainsharing. As you look into developing a total compensation system that's best for your practice, recognize that performance pay plans should reflect organizational goals and values and enhance your performance management system. If you have the commitment and resources to do it the right way, strategically designed pay is a powerful tool for aligning individual and practice performance, and for ensuring that employee contributions are rewarded.

References:

1. Janet Wiscombe, "Can Pay for Performance Really Work?" www.workforce.com, 2001.

2. "Employee Management," *An Assessment Manual for Medical Groups,* MGMA, Denver, CO, 2002.

3. Gordon W. Hawthorne and C.J. Bolster, "10th Annual Compensation and Salary Guide," Health & Health Networks Magazine, www.hhnmag.com.

4. Valerie L. Williams and Stephen E. Grimaldi, "Fundamental Elements of a Total Compensation System," www.workforce.com.

5. Todd Raphael, "Employees in Every Industry Watch Hospitals' Staffing Solutions," www.workforce.com, 2001.

6. Todd Raphael, "Employees in Every Industry Watch Hospitals' Staffing Solutions," www.workforce.com, 2001.

7. Valerie L. Williams and Stephen E. Grimaldi, "Fundamental Elements of a Total Compensation System," www.workforce.com.

8. "Switch to Production Pay Plan Brightens Bottom Line for Groups," Inside PPMCs, February 2, 2000, vol. 4, No.3, pp. 1-6.

9. "Quality, Often Avoided as Pay Factor, Can improve Marketing and Incomes, Physician Compensation Report, April 12, 2000.

10. Janet Wiscombe, "Can Pay for Performance Really Work?" Workforce, August 2001, pp. 28-34.

11. Anntoinette D. Lucia, HR Magazine, January 2000, p. 142, excerpted from, *The Art and Science of Competency Models: Pinpointing Critical Success Factors in Organizations,* San Francisco, CA, Jossey-Bass/Pfeiffer, 1999.

12. Anntoinette D. Lucia, HR Magazine, January 2000, p. 142, excerpted from, *The Art and Science of Competency Models: Pinpointing Critical Success Factors in Organizations,* San Francisco, CA, Jossey-Bass/Pfeiffer, 1999.

13. Joseph H. Boyett and Jimmie T. Boyett, *Pay for Knowledge Design Workbook,* Alpharetta, GA, Boyett & Associates, 2000.

14. Lyle M. Spencer and Signe M. Spencer, *Competence at Work: Models for Superior Performance*, John Wiley & Sons, 1993.

15. Lyle M. Spencer and Signe M. Spencer, *Competence at Work: Models for Superior Performance,* John Wiley & Sons, 1993.

16. Anntoinette D. Lucia, HR Magazine, January 2000, p. 142, excerpted from, *The Art and Science of Competency Models: Pinpointing Critical Success Factors in Organizations,* San Francisco, CA, Jossey-Bass/Pfeiffer, 1999.

17. Joseph H. Boyett and Jimmie T. Boyett, *The Gainsharing Workbook,* Alpharetta, GA, Boyett & Associates, 1999.

18. John Washlick, Esq., "Physician-Hospital Gainsharing Arrangements," Physicians News Digest, October 1999.

19. *Health & Health Care 2010: The Forecast, the Challenge, Institute for the Future,* Menlo Park, CA, www.iftf.org, 2000 excerpted from The Compensation Monitor, April 2000.

The Role of Rewards and Recognition

Chapter 7

"Just as the accumulation of small improvements can make a dramatic, lasting change in the organization's products or services, the repeated, numerous small occasions of taking note of the contributions of individuals and teams of individuals can create a different company."[1]

-Patrick Townsend and Joan Gebhardt

Reward and recognition programs are an essential component of every successful practice. Studies indicate that praise, rewards and recognition can motivate employees to put forth their best efforts and perform at higher levels. Everyone wants to be appreciated for doing a good job. The purpose of employee recognition and rewards can be to recognize achievement of a specific performance goal; or just to say "thank you," "you're doing a great job," "we value you." Recognition is different than other types of compensation such as salary, which is payment for performing the job, or benefits, which are to safeguard the employee's well being. To be successful, a reward program must be customized to fit your practice's culture.[2]

In this chapter, you'll explore best practices in offering recognition and rewards as part of your performance management system. Specifically, you will review:

- Innovative guidelines for giving recognition and rewards;

- Best practices – types of recognition and rewards; and
- Success guidelines for implementing a recognition program for star performers.

For additional information on reward programs for medical practices including incentive pay, combination rewards, physician performance rewards and more, reference *The Medical Practice Performance Management Manual: How To Evaluate Employees*, pages 191-202.

Guidelines for Giving Recognition and Rewards

According to Bob Nelson, the author of *1001 Ways to Reward Employees,* the concept of positive reinforcement or rewarding behavior that you want to see repeated truly works. As a supervisor or manager, it is your responsibility to set the example of actively appreciating employee efforts and rewarding for results. For example, it is just as important to recognize a team or individual when they accomplish a milestone or come close to a meeting a goal rather than just appreciating them when they reach it. This technique will motivate the team to persist toward the desired results.

As noted in a book excerpt from CIO magazine[3], top performers represent only 10 percent of your workforce. It is the other 90 percent of your workforce who will benefit the most from receiving positive reinforcement and incentives along the way in order to achieve top performance and repeat outstanding performance. This is why it is crucial to use rewards and recognition to impact performance and get the results desired.

Appreciation and recognition are instrumental in bringing out the best in people, yet most managers and supervisors fail to understand or use this potential power. The typical reason that managers do not use recognition as a performance motivator is because they believe only monetary forms of recognition such as raises or promotions are appreciated. While money is important to employees, a survey conducted by Watson Wyatt Worldwide[4] showed that employers are offering more non-monetary incentives to motivate employees such as:

- Advancement opportunities;
- Flexible work schedules;
- Opportunities to learn new skills;
- Career development;
- Telecommuting;
- Reduced work weeks;
- Job redesign; and
- Sabbaticals.

Furthermore, thoughtful, personal recognition that doesn't cost a lot of money but gives the employee a story to tell to family and friends can make a lasting impression on employees for years.[5] Examples of personal recognition rewards will be discussed later in this chapter.

The following list provides some effective guidelines that can help to teach you the essential elements of good recognition. Keep these guidelines in mind each time you recognize your employee for doing a good job or giving 110 percent!

Innovative Guidelines for Giving Recognition and Rewards

1. Timely
2. Specific
3. Genuine
4. Equivalent
5. Meaningful
6. Motivational

Timely Make sure that recognition happens as close to the event or behavior as possible. When you hear a good word about an employee from a patient or co-worker, make sure you thank the employee for his or her good work as soon as possible. If you wait too long to recognize your employee, it loses all of its value and motivational effect.

Specific Explain to employees why they are being recognized giving detailed examples of behavior. For example, you could say to your employee, "Jane, I want to let you know that three patients have personally commented to me about your pleasant and professional manner on the phone. I want to thank you for providing outstanding service to our customers and helping make this practice stand out!" This will help the employee to understand exactly what behavior or action you would like to continue

Genuine Be sincere in your praise or recognition for an employee. When you are happy with employee performance, show it with your body language, actions and words. Smile, shake their hands, and be genuinely excited for them. If at all possible, always give recognition face to face because it makes the recognition more personal and the employee can clearly see your reaction. Remember, if your employees are doing a great job, it will have a reflection on you and the entire practice.

Equivalent Make sure that the reward matches the level of the achievement or performance goal. For example, an employee who completes a two-year project should be rewarded in a more substantial way than someone who filled in for a sick employee at the last minute. The more important the achievement, the larger the recognition or reward should be.

Meaningful Find out what is important to your employees including what hobbies they enjoy so that you can recognize them in a way that is "special" and meaningful to them. For example, some employees may want personal recognition done in private; some may enjoy gifts or other tangible items; while other employees may view advanced training for their career development as a very motivational reward.

Motivational Make sure that employees are feeling motivated to perform at higher levels by your recognition and reward efforts. One way to ensure that your rewards are going to motivate employees is to involve them in determining the types of recognition and rewards offered. If employees are not excited when they receive a reward and good performance is not continuing, then it may be time to rethink your program and come up with some new ideas.

Source: Powers, Tara, Powers Training & Developmental Resources, 2001.

Types of Recognition and Rewards

1. Incentives
2. Service Awards
3. Personal Recognition for:
   - Individuals
   - Co-workers
   - Teams
   - Organization- wide
4. Star Performer Rewards

Types of Recognition and Rewards

To repeat the maxim of this book: The most valuable asset in any group practice is the people who work there. One of the most important ways to increase the value of that asset is to appreciate your employees for a job well done. Recognition and rewards can come in a variety of styles, values and awards. Keep in mind that positive reinforcement stands for whatever a person will work hard to get. This does not always have to include money but could be as simple as a smile, a thank you, or even a handwritten note. Some of the most meaningful forms of recognition can cost nothing at all.

When designing any type of recognition or reward program, keep in mind the different generations in your practice and what they might value as a reward.[6]

For example, *veterans,* who value tradition and hard work, enjoy personal and symbolic recognition such as:

- A simple thank you
- A handwritten note
- A plaque or certificate
- Any recognition that is more personal and face to face

On the other hand, *baby boomers* who thrive on working their way to the top, are team players and value a strong work ethic, prefer:

- Lots of public recognition
- Company perks, cars, trips, etc.
- Getting name recognition throughout the company
- Recognition for working long hours

G*enerations Xers* who have a "work to live" mentality, enjoy a casual and comfortable workplace and are savvy with computers, prefer:

- Empowerment. Give your employees the opportunity to work on a new project and make decisions on their own
- Flexible work schedules
- Shortened work weeks
- Telecommuting
- Opportunity to work with leading edge technology

Reasons To Use Incentives

1. Efficiency
2. Customer Service
3. Motivation
4. Retention
5. Measurement

Lastly, *Generation Y,* the newest group to reach the workforce is interested in recognition that includes:

- Training and career development opportunities;
- Money for advanced degrees; and
- Opportunities to work on team projects.

Incentives

According to an article by Susan Marks in Workforce Magazine, incentives are essential in keeping top performers satisfied with their overall compensation packages. "Businesses cannot afford to have their most talented employees jump ship," says Frank Belmonte, HR consultant and principal with Hewitt Associates LLC, global management consultants.[7]

Incentives can be in cash, performance-based pay or bonuses. Incentives can also be cash equivalents like travel awards, or other benefits such as offering employee training, which is a powerful retention tool used by many companies.

Reasons To Use Incentives In Your Practice

1. ***Improve Efficiency.*** As noted earlier, 90 percent of your workforce is comprised of "average achievers." This group needs a little extra push to improve their productivity and efficiency in the office. Incentives are strategies designed to effectively push this 90 percent a little harder.

2. ***Improve Customer Service.*** First impressions begin with the type of service customers get from the moment they walk into your practice or make a call on the telephone. It is imperative to ensure the employees who are generating these first impressions are patient, friendly and knowledgeable. Offering incentives for improved customer satisfaction can have a large impact on the level of customer service in your practice.

3. ***As a Motivational Tool.*** New policies or procedures often are communicated to employees through training but rarely include follow-up to ensure implementation. When introducing employees to a new procedure or product, consider offering rewards that relate to the

training process. Items such as pens, T-shirts or mouse pads can be used as encouragement to implement what they have learned and are relatively inexpensive. Any type of incentive that can be offered year-round can promote camaraderie and increase employee morale.

4. ***As a Retention Tool.*** It is more difficult than ever to find and retain star employees. If your practice has an incentive program and you actively appreciate your employees for their hard work, you will fare much better in retention than other practices that simply overlook employee contributions.

5. ***Measurement.*** Incentives can be a great way to measure progress in your practice. By offering different levels of rewards at milestone achievements, managers will have a good indication of where their employees stand. [7]

How To Develop an Incentive Program

1. Determine Objectives.
2. Plan a Strategy.
3. Define Measurement.
4. Have a Budget.
5. Choose Rewards.
6. Implement Program.
7. Celebrate Success.
8. Evaluate.

How to Develop an Incentive Program

1. ***Determine Objectives.*** Identify what needs to be accomplished such as better attendance, improved customer service, healthier communication, more efficient decision-making, increased teamwork, etc. Keep your objectives simple, specific and achievable. Make sure that the objective is stated and communicated to all employees involved in program.

   Example: This practice has seen a decrease in communication between the staff over the past six months. This has caused an increase in paperwork not being processed correctly due to misunderstanding and lack of information. Examples include claims not being sent in on time, patient files not being updated, prescriptions not being called in to the pharmacies in a timely manner. The goal is to get the staff working together on a daily basis, sharing information and resources to reduce costly errors to the practice.

2. **Plan a Strategy.** Define length of the program, when the program will begin, how incentives will be used, who will be involved, and what effect success will have on the practice.

Example: We will work on increasing communication throughout this fiscal year. This is a top priority for the practice this year. Incentives will be rewarded to employees who help the practice meet its goal by offering new ideas for improving communication and ensuring the successful implementation of those ideas. If the staff can learn to communicate effectively with one another on a regular basis, the practice should experience fewer errors and consequently be more profitable for the year.

3. ***Define Measurement.*** Once objectives have been defined, clearly state how they will be measured. How will you know when you have achieved the objectives? What will success look like?

   Example: The goal of improving communication among the staff will be measured by taking a look at statistical information from last year and comparing it to this year. Focus on the following areas:

   - errors in patient paperwork;
   - customer complaints; and
   - number of claims that have to be reprocessed.

   The practice wants to see at least a 10 percent decrease in the areas listed to consider the goal a success.

4. ***Create and Manage a Budge***t. Create a budget for any type of reward program. Items to consider when budgeting include:

   - number of employees involved;
   - range of rewards that you choose and their associated cost;
   - how long program will last;
   - administration time and cost; and
   - expected results.

   Example: The practice has established a budget for implementing ideas to meet the goal. Each employee will be able to choose two training sessions dealing with communication skills that they would like to attend during the year as well as having an off-site team retreat in

March. Any employee who has an idea to improve communication can bring it up at the weekly staff meeting and everyone can vote on it to decide if it will be implemented.

5. **Choose Rewards.** Spend time talking with employees and teams to find out what is important to them and what they value. This can be done in weekly staff meetings, surveys, one-on-one conversations or by distributing a "What's your preference" sheet. A supervisor can distribute a brief questionnaire to employees to find out what they value and appreciate.

   For example, a short questionnaire to employees might include questions like:

   - What are your hobbies or interests? (i.e., art, horses, old cars)
   - What is your favorite activity? (i.e., boating, fishing, skiing, hiking)
   - What do you like to do when you have time off from work? (i.e., spend time with kids, go to the movies, take a trip)
   - What small type of reward (under $100) would you enjoy receiving? (i.e., concert tickets, massage, dinner at favorite restaurant)
   - What do you think would be a good team award? (i.e., group outing, catered lunch)

   Remember: If employees are not motivated to obtain the reward, they will not pursue the goal

   Example: Based on the employee survey that was sent out, the practice has developed the following rewards and incentives for meeting the goal:

   - Any employee who suggests a new communication tool for the team that is implemented will receive a weekend for two at a ski resort.

6. **Implement the Program.** Employees should now have a clear understanding of the goal, the incentive and the expected outcome. The supervisor can officially kick off the program by announcing it at a staff meeting, hanging up posters, or initiating other creative ideas to get employees excited about reaching the goal!

Example: "Operation Communication" was engraved on pencils, pens and sticky notes and distributed to all employees. This provided employees with a constant reminder of the importance of reaching this goal by the end of the year.

7. **Celebrate Success.** Once employees have reached their goal or objective, celebrate! Hold a luncheon, picnic, catered dinner or impromptu party. Clearly articulate to all employees the achievement and its impact on the practice. Individuals or teams should then receive their rewards.

   Example: "Operation Communication" was a success and all employees were invited to celebrate at a local restaurant for Happy Hour. Once all employees arrived, the supervisor discussed how communication had improved by using the measurements that were in place. Employees who came up with communication tools that were implemented were given their reward and each staff member was rewarded a "weekend of fun and sun" with four free passes to the local theme park to use with their families.

8. **Evaluate.** Did the incentive program achieve its objectives based on the measures that were defined earlier in the program? Did the participants change their behavior? Remember, incentives aim at short-term objectives so follow-up and evaluation is very important. New incentives will need to be implemented periodically. [8]

Service Awards

Longevity and loyalty with your practice should be rewarded and recognized. Effective service award programs should make employees feel that management cares about them as individuals and truly values their years of hard work and commitment to the practice. Service rewards should represent something meaningful to the employees that signifies their contribution and service.

Examples of service rewards will vary in cost and significance depending on the years of service. Some suggestions are:

- 1-5 years:
  - Plaques
  - Pins
  - Engraved pens
  - Banquet for employees
- 5-10 years:
  - Jewelry
  - Watches
  - Crystal sculptures engraved with number of years of service
  - Banquet with Board of Directors
  - Shares of stock
  - Paid vacation

When thinking about meaningful service rewards for your employees, keep in mind that baby boomers usually like to be recognized incrementally for their years of service where as Generation X employees prefer personal, practical rewards such as grills, bicycles or even trips.[9]

Caution: Once you have designed a service award program, if your employees start asking for cash in lieu of the award or say that they don't want the award, it means your program isn't working. This should prompt you to take another look at the rewards you are offering because they are probably not meeting your objectives of being meaningful and valuable to your employees.

Personal Recognition

Personal recognition can be very informal and inexpensive for your practice to implement. Sincere and appropriate recognition at the right time and the right place can mean more to an employee than money, bonuses or bunch of certificates. The power of "Thank You" should never be overlooked.

Types of personal recognition could include:[10]

- **Individual** recognition where the manager provides recognition based on individual achievements. This is a critical component of performance management and feedback.

- **Co-worker to co-worker** recognition that builds on teamwork, communication and cooperation among co-workers.
- **Team** recognition which supports and encourages team performance.
- **Organization-wid**e recognition for the entire practice or organization in meeting its strategic objectives, surpassing revenue and income projections or being recognized as industry leaders.

Individual Recognition

"Verbal praise from one's manager is a top motivator for employees; it's consistently ranked high in surveys of workplace motivators."[10]

- Bob Nelson

In Bob Nelson's book *1001 Ways to Reward Employees,* he suggests three simple ways for a manager to recognize an employee.[10]

1. **To Their Face** – Go up to an employee and recognize him or her face-to-face as soon as an achievement or desired behavior has taken place. Make sure to explain in detail why the employee is being recognized and show how the employee's achievement will help the entire practice.

2. **In Front of Co-workers or Peers** – Recognizing employees in front of their co-workers can be a very powerful and unforgettable experience for an employee. This could be done at a staff meeting, in the lunchroom, or even in the hallway!

3. **When the Employee is NOT present** – If you recognize employees when they are not present, you can bet that your words of praise will quickly be communicated to the person you were speaking of. Employees see this as one of the most powerful forms of recognition a manager can give

Other individual awards include:

On-the-spot awards - which can be given at a moment's notice to any employee who has gone "above and beyond the call of duty." Possibly your employee filled in for someone at a moment's notice; someone came in to work on the weekend to finish a big project; or another took on additional responsibility without complaining because you are short-staffed. These rewards usually focus on a one-time achievement and are given on the spot once the achievement is realized. Keep in mind that a reward you know your employee will value will have a greater impact than giving all your employees the same reward time and time again.

Examples:

- movie tickets
- theatre tickets
- grocery certificates
- gift certificates to play a round of golf
- concert tickets
- day off of work
- gift certificate to a spa
- gift certificate to company store
- "night on the town" award where company reimburses employee for a night out of dinner, dancing and movie

Co-worker to Co-worker Recognition

Many employees consider peer recognition one of the most meaningful forms of recognition they can receive. Managers and supervisors are critical in setting the example for this type of recognition between employees. By involving employees in recognizing their team members or co-workers, it creates commitment to recognition as well as buy-in to the program.[10]

One of the simplest and most effective ways to promote peer recognition is allowing employees to recognize their peers whose efforts are outstanding as part of weekly staff meetings.

Other ideas to assist you in helping your employees recognize one another could include:

- Recognize outstanding skill or expertise by allowing an employee to mentor another.
- Start a traveling trophy award (make it original) – this award can be passed on from person to person for developing a creative idea or a better way to do something! One example is the "kick butt" award symbolized by a

cowboy boot passed around from co-worker to co-worker when someone has done an outstanding job.

- Explain to employees the important of recognition and get them involved in praising one another in front of co-workers, strangers or customers.
- Develop a "Pass It On" card and every few months hand these out at a departmental staff meeting. Tell employees they have 48 hours to give this card to someone whom they work with who has made some difference in their lives.[11]

Team Recognition

The first step managers should take in using recognition to build a high performing team is to acknowledge the successes of all team members. Some of the best forms of team recognition are personal, such as the manager individually thanking each member of the team who has done a good job; thanking group members for their involvement, suggestions and initiative; or sending a letter to all team members thanking them for their contributions.[12]

Be creative! Managers and supervisors should remember that simpler ideas are easier to implement and they don't need to be elaborate to be effective. Ideas could range from the CEO coming to the team meeting to thank the team for a job well done, to team logos on T-shirts, mugs or hats to catered breakfasts or lunches. Gift certificates to a spa after working on a big project or taking the team out for dinner and movie are some other good suggestions. Whatever you decide, team recognition should be personal and simple. Remember, team accomplishments are valued by the entire organization; they can boost morale and commitment among a larger group of employees. When a team is recognized, they feel a sense of group accomplishment and satisfaction that they collectively reached a goal or milestone. This sense of "teamwork" differs from individual recognition but is just as important.

Organization-Wide

Recognition for the organization is necessary anytime there is a big win, organizational goals have been accomplished or revenue has exceeded expectations. When organizational success is achieved, it is by the commitment and perseverance of all employees. Therefore, to recognize the organization and all who have made it successful, a reward needs to include all employees. Some organization-wide recognition ideas:

- Company picnic
- Banquet
- Catered dinner
- Ball game
- Ski Day
- Family day at the zoo or local museum
- Keynote speaker at company-wide event
- Company party

Star Performer Rewards

Most organizations have an outstanding employee or employee of the month award that recognizes top performers. This type of award can be given for a single exceptional achievement such as catching a $20,000 dollar mistake or coming up with an idea that saved the organization thousands of dollars, or it could be for a multitude of recognizable achievements such as numerous compliments from customers, or completion of many outstanding projects.

What makes a star performer reward memorable is when peers and co-workers are involved in the selection process as well as management. Make sure all employees know how and why an employee can receive the star performer award. These details and decisions should be decided on by all employees in a group staff meeting. Employees can then nominate a star performer by sending an e-mail to management when they feel someone is deserving of the award. The e-mail will need to detail the specifics of why they deserve the award and examples of what they have done to support it.

Star performer rewards should be meaningful and personal, based on what the employee values most. The cost of the reward will depend on the organization's budget. Ideas for the star performer award could include:

- A family vacation
- Free daycare for the month
- A shopping spree at employee's favorite store

- Lunch with the president of the company
- $100 savings bond
- Reserved parking space for the month

Evaluating Recognition

If you want to find out if your employees are being motivated by your recognition efforts, just ask them. It is important to find out how employees feel about the recognition ideas that your practice has decided to implement. Most organizations with recognition programs in place send out short satisfaction surveys every six months to make sure the program is still working and motivating employees to perform.

Feedback from employees can provide information for continued support or changes to the program to make it successful. Simple attitude surveys can reveal your employees' reactions to the recognition ideas your department has implemented. Following are a few sample questions from such a survey.

Employee Survey

- ❏ I feel that I am recognized for the good work that I do by my manager? Why or why not?
- ❏ Are you appreciated for the work you do? Please give three examples.
- ❏ How does your team or department make you feel like you are a valuable contributor to the medical practice?
- ❏ Please explain how and why employees get recognized at work.
- ❏ Is recognition in this group practice fair and consistent? Why or why not?
- ❏ I like the recognition and rewards provided by the practice? Yes? No? Why?
- ❏ Please provide suggestions for improvement.

Guidelines for Implementing an Effective Recognition Program

If you are interested in implementing recognition and rewards in your practice, the following guidelines provide information on how to get started:

✓ Any reward or recognition program should be in-line with the mission, values and business strategies of the practice.
✓ Employees should be able to participate in developing a program. When employees are involved in developing the recognition program, they will be motivated to participate and ensure its success.
✓ Be clear on the program objectives so that all employees understand why rewards are given.
✓ Define what constitutes receiving a reward. For example, what do you have to do to receive the star performer award?
✓ Reward should involve the use of cash, non-cash or both and should be considered something of value by employees.
✓ Have a variety of resources and tools to use. There are many companies listed on the Internet that work with organizations to develop reward programs. They also have great suggestions for reward ideas. Some resources are:

- www.Nelson-motivation.com
- www.recognition.org
- www.giftcertificates.com
- www.incentivemarketing.org

✓ Everyone in the practice should be aware of the program. Hang up posters, pass out flyers, make sure everyone knows about your recognition program
✓ Rewards will need to be evaluated over time to decide if they need to be updated or changed. Survey employees every six months to make sure your program is still working.
✓ Rewards and recognition should be "matched" to employee preferences and to the achievement. The bigger the achievement, the bigger the reward should be. [13]

Summary

In summary, recognition and rewards are an integral part of an effective performance management system. Employees are looking for a sense of recognition, status, achievement, respect and self-fulfillment. When you understand and meet these higher level needs of your employees, you help them to develop to their full potential. Recognition and rewards don't have to be expensive and certainly any investment is less than the cost of recruiting and training a new employee. The ideas for recognition are endless and many of them can come from your employees and managers.

References

1. Bob Nelson, *1001 Ways To Reward Employees,* Workman Publishing Company, New York, 1994.
2. P. Schiffers, S. Young, D. Shelton, "Employee Recognition and Reward Programs That Work", http://www.shrm.org/whitepapers, October 1996.
3. "STAR makers" CIO Magazine, September 2000, p.226.
4. "Playing to Win: Strategic Rewards in the War for Talent", Wyatt Watson Fifth Annual Survey Report 2000/2001, http://vault.com/nr/printable.jsp?ch_id=253&article_id=1809301&print=1
5. Bob Nelson, *1001 Ways To Reward Employees,* Workman Publishing Company, New York, 1994.
6. Ron Zemke, Claire Raines, Bob Filipczak, *Generations At Work*, Amacom, 2000.
7. Susan J. Marks, "Incentives That Really Reward and Motivate" Workforce, June 2001, pg 108.
8. P. Schiffers, S. Young, D. Shelton, "Employee Recognition and Reward Programs That Work", http://www.shrm.org/whitepapers, October 1996.
9. Ron Zemke, Claire Raines, Bob Filipczak, *Generations At Work*, Amacom, 2000.
10. Bob Nelson, *1001 Ways To Reward Employees,* Workman Publishing Company, New York, 1994.
11. Barbara A. Glanz, *Care Packages For The Workplace,* McGraw Hill, New York, 1995.
12. Bob Nelson, "Seven Ways To Praise Teams" Workforce, February, 1997
13. Bob Nelson, *1001 Ways To Reward Employees,* Workman Publishing Company, New York, 1994.

Additional Resources:

http://www.therobbinsco.com/sollib_source/10_reasons.html

http://www.incentivemarketing.org/IndustryResearch.html

Ensuring Successful Integration

Chapter 8

"The best organizations create performance management systems that are as Einstein said, the solution to any problem should be as simple as possible or simpler...They identify the competencies that are keen to the organization's overall success and demand that everyone be held accountable for performing like a master...Finally, they closely link their performance system with their strategy, mission statement, and vision and values..."

-Dick Grote, Grote Consulting Corporation[1]

By now you have an understanding of the components of a performance management system and how to implement each component. What are the other factors to ensure that your system will be embraced and used effectively in the group practice?

This chapter explores six critical areas for integration and ongoing management that are vital if your performance management system is to be anchored and developed successfully: (1) introducing new hires to the performance management system; (2) using proper documentation techniques; (3) training supervisors and other key people; (4) evaluating and revising your system; (5) using online performance management systems; and (6) legal caution. Understanding each of these critical areas and how they can impact your performance management system before, during and after integration will save you time, resources and legal challenges.

Five Reasons Why Orientation is Critical

1. Start-up costs
2. Anxiety
3. Employee turnover
4. Time
5. Role expectations

Introducing New Hires to the Performance Management System

There are several reasons why medical group practices should provide an orientation for new hires. Although orientation may seem like a celebratory event and a "waste of time and productivity" for managers and staff members, resources have indicated that orientation (or lack of it) will make a significant difference in how quickly new employees become productive. It will have long-term effects on organizations. [2]

There are five reasons why your group practice should properly introduce your new hires to the organization, other employees, and particularly to the performance management system in place:

1. *To reduce start-up costs*—Proper orientation can help employees get "up to speed" quicker, reducing the costs associated with learning new roles.
2. *To reduce anxiety*—All new employees experience anxiety when put into a new situation or position. A proper orientation not only reduces anxiety, it also provides guidelines for performance behavior and culture.
3. *To reduce employee turnover*—Most turnover with new hires occurs because they don't feel valued or are placed in positions where they don't think they'll be successful. Orientation can help provide necessary tools and guidelines to perform a job effectively.
4. *To save time for co-workers and supervisors*—The better the orientation, the less likely new hires will require as much training to get started. This saves time and resources for the practice.
5. *To develop realistic expectations about roles*—New employees should learn from the start what is expected of them, what to expect from co-workers, managers and supervisors, as well as the values and goals of the practice.

Overview Orientation

Many organizations provide two kinds of orientation: an Overview Orientation that provides basic information about the medical group practice and the broader system that employees work in. This kind of orientation may be provided by the personnel department, an office manager or supervisor and generally includes information about:

- History and background information of the organization;
- Important policies and procedures that are non-job specific;
- Compensation philosophy and benefits;
- Safety and accident prevention guidelines; and
- Physical facilities.

Job-Specific Orientation

The second kind of new hire orientation is often job-specific and helps new employees to understand:

- How the employee fits into the overall organization;
- Job responsibilities, expectations and duties;
- Policies, procedures, rules and regulations;
- Layout of workspace and personal office area, as appropriate; and
- Introduction to co-workers and key people in their work area.

The new employee's manager or supervisor best provides this kind of orientation. Many times, this orientation is ongoing with other co-workers and supervisors supplying coaching.[3] Consider assigning a new employee a buddy or mentor. It should preferably be someone the new employee would have a lot of contact with over the first two or three months. This person can provide a constant resource for information, guidance and learning.

Another important reason to provide an orientation for new hires is that legally, some type of orientation must take place. Otherwise, a new employee could actually sue the group practice for wrongful misrepresentation or wrongful hiring. Employers are obligated to provide a clear, specific, accurate representation of the position, salary, location and responsibilities before a job offer is made. If all of this information is not provided prior to the start date, employees should receive necessary information on the first day.

The best way to enroll employees into your performance management system is to introduce them to it from the start and help them to be successful at meeting their objectives early in their employment.[4]

Three Reasons to Document Performance

1. Performance improvement
2. Personnel decisions
3. Lawsuit protection

Using Proper Documentation Techniques

Maintaining accurate, complete and current documentation for employee performance is important for managers and supervisors to evaluate performance fairly and consistently. Performance should be documented in your practice for three main reasons:

1. To improve or maintain good performance.
2. To support personnel decisions.
3. To protect your practice from lawsuits as a result of making personnel decisions.

One of the best ways to document employee performance is to use a performance journal. A performance journal like the model provided in Figure 8-1 should be used on a consistent basis for each employee. It should be easy to access and utilize, providing just enough details to remember what happened and when. Should an employee's performance become an issue, this journal can serve as a record of what steps managers and supervisors took to address and resolve the problem.

A performance journal should be created and maintained for each direct report. It can easily be created and maintained on your computer using a word processor or as simple as using a tablet for each employee and writing entries as needed. For those interested in using an electronic format, review the information provided later in this chapter in the section entitled, "Using Online Performance Management Systems."

Using a Performance Journal

Managers and supervisors should develop a habit of keeping a journal or record of key events related to employee performance. Keep in mind that the positive reason entries are made is because your practice wants an employee to succeed in his or her job. "Secret" notes like those thought to be in a "black book" are inappropriate. If something is important enough to write down, it's important enough to discuss with the employee.[5]

Key events to record in an performance journal are things like:

✓ Goal setting conversations;
✓ Formal conversations about job responsibilities or projects;
✓ Counseling, coaching or delegating sessions;
✓ Recognition for good work;
✓ Customer complaints and compliments;
✓ Examples of poor or outstanding work;
✓ Attendance issues; and
✓ Disciplinary actions.

What to Record

- **Setting Goals, Objectives or Expectations** – make a journal entry any time you discuss and agree upon goals, objectives or job expectations with your employees. It is helpful to include dates and also the goal or expectation the employee has agreed to meet.
- **Recognition** – note if an employee goes above and beyond what is expected or consistently meets objectives and expectations.
- **Training** – note any employee training that took place, both on-the-job training and professional development courses.
- **Coaching/Counseling** – note any employee coaching/counseling sessions as they occur. This demonstrates that the supervisor worked with the employee to resolve a problem in its early stages or to help an employee improve his or her performance.
- **Investigations** – anytime an investigation takes place information should be recorded to help remember conversations and what was said.

- **Progressive Discipline** – note each step of progressive discipline taken in the performance journal.

Documenting Poor Performance

- Record facts that define the performance problem.
- Record explanations to the employee on role expectations.
- Describe solutions that can help the employee meet performance objectives.
- State actions that will take place if the problem is not corrected.

Documenting Poor Performance

When documenting poor performance or progressive discipline issues, use the following guidelines to make documentation in performance journal, managers' or supervisors' notes or in employees' personnel files. By using these steps and following a consistent format, managers and supervisors can help employees with performance problems and comply with legal documentation requirements.[5]

Record facts *that define the problem*

- **What** happened;
- **When** it happened;
- **Where** it happened;
- **Who** was involved; and
- **Why** it happened.

Record explanations *to the employee on the expectations of his or her role:*

- Define what the employee must accomplish to meet performance expectations.
- Indicate why the employee's performance is important to the practice.
- Clarify the results to be achieved.
- State the measurable outcomes expected.

Describe solutions *that can help the employee meet performance objectives.*

- Offer employee training in the area that needs to be improved.
- Tell the employee how he or she can be successful in meeting expectations.
- Offer options the employee could take to resolve the problem.
- Give suggested course of actions.
- Document any ideas you gave the employee as a solution to improving his or her performance.

State actions *that will take place if the problem is not corrected.*

- Document the action you intend to take if the employee does not meet performance objectives.
- Clearly communicate further actions and consequences to the employee.
- Declare the seriousness of the situation.
- Offer your commitment to helping the employee resolve the problem.
- Make sure the employee understands his or her job is in jeopardy.

The performance journal will allow managers and supervisors to maintain all entries specific to an employee. A sample performance journal reflecting various types of entries is provided in Figure 8-1.

Figure 8-1
Sample Performance Journal

Susie Smith

Thursday, January 15
Counseling Session

11:00 a.m. I witnessed Susie yell at a patient this morning. Asked her why. She said it was because she was having problems at home. She has agreed to use our Employee Assistance Program. She understands that this is her first warning. We decided to meet again in two weeks to discuss how things are going.

Tuesday, February 1
Written Warning/Suspension

1:00 p.m. Susie yelled at a patient today who forgot his checkbook. I sent her home without pay for the remainder of the day. I requested that Susie seriously consider whether she wants to continue working at our office and to return with a written explanation of what she can and will do to improve her customer service skills immediately. Susie understands that if this happens again she may be terminated. Gave her a copy of the written warning memo and placed copy in her personnel file. Susie signed the original.

Wednesday, March 5
Positive Feedback
8:30 a.m. Ms. Wright called me this morning to compliment on Susie's professional and pleasant demeanor when handling her requests for her patient history records. I recognized Susie in front of her co-workers and complimented her on her customer service skills. Susie has shown great improvement in this area.

Seven Steps for Informal Actions

1. Discuss situation.
2. Explain performance expectation.
3. Get agreement.
4. Explore steps.
5. Ask about action.
6. Discuss consequences.
7. Promise feedback.

Taking Action for Performance Improvement

Once poor performance has been documented, managers and supervisors should bring the issue to the employee's attention as soon as possible. By identifying, communicating and addressing performance issues, an employee is more likely to improve his or her performance. Remember, effective performance management offers timely action to have the best outcomes. Most practices use both informal and formal actions to address performance issues with employees.

Informal Actions

Informal actions are most appropriate when minor performance issues arise; when it's apparent that it's the first time an employee has needed intervention; or if there may be a mismatch in skills and abilities. Your practice may find that a coaching or counseling session with the employee is all it takes to address the issue. Using these steps will help make the session more effective:

1. Discuss the situation with the employee.
2. Explain what the performance expectation is and show how the employee isn't meeting it.
3. The employee should agree, or at least understand, that he or she is accountable for meeting this expectation.
4. Jointly explore steps or solutions to ensure that the expectation will be met.
5. Ask the employee how he or she plans to meet expectation or standard. If the employee is unable to offer any suggestions, you should make some suggestions. It's critical that the employee owns the solution and is committed to improve the deficiency.
6. Discuss possible consequences if the issue can't be resolved.
7. Let the employee know how and when you'll follow up with additional feedback.

Formal Action Steps

Step 1: Verbal Reminder
Step 2: Written Reminder
Step 3: Final Warning

Formal Actions

Formal actions should be documented and addressed in a different way. These actions are generally taken because of repeated problems or performance issues that are more serious. If performance issues do not improve, it may be necessary to consider disciplinary action or termination.

Step One–Verbal Reminder
Similar to the coaching and counseling session for an informal action. In addition, the manager or supervisor indicates that this is a verbal warning and may have additional consequences if the issue is not resolved.

Step Two—Written Reminder
If after an oral warning has been provided to the employee and performance has not improved, a written reminder is given. During this session, remind the employee of the prior discussion and that the commitments were not met. The manager or supervisor should try to get the employee's commitment to resolve the problem. Consequences for not improving performance should be stated and the employee must be told that this is second warning. An action plan should be agreed to with follow-up actions and timelines.

"This sometimes works better than immediately issuing a disciplinary notice. It puts the employee on notice that you are serious when you ask for improvement in performance, and it documents the discussion." —Mary Cook, 2001[6]

HR experts recommend giving employees opportunities to improve their performance before taking further disciplinary action. One way of doing this is by creating a written performance improvement plan with the employee and using the plan as a guide to monitor improvement. Mary Cook, the author of, *The Complete Do-It-Yourself Human Resources Department* (2001) suggests using a consistent format for this plan. It can be as simple as a memo that states the performance issue, the steps taken such as verbal warning, and the expectations for improvement. Also be sure to note the consequences if improvement does not occur within a specific time frame. Both the supervisor and employee should sign and date the document.

Step Three—Final Warning

If performance does not improve to the level necessary to meet the practice's expectations, a final warning is given to the employee.[7]

An example of a final warning is provided in Figure 8-2. Notice how the manager cites each incident, the verbal warning step, and the possible consequences that may be considered if the employee's chronic absenteeism continues. This type of documentation in essential when disciplinary action is likely to follow.

Figure 8-2
Sample Performance Memo:
Poor Customer Service

To: Susie Smith
From: Jane Doe, Manager
Date: February 2, 2002
RE: Written Warning

On January 15, 25 and February 1, you were observed by fellow co-workers and by myself yelling at our patients in the office. Our policy states: "It is our responsibility and duty to treat each patient with care and respect." Each of these instances took place after having a conversation with your husband on the telephone. On January 15, I counseled you about your attitude and demeanor toward our patients and gave you a verbal warning. You stated that you were having problems at home and agreed to use our Employee Assistance Program. On January 25 you were overheard telling a patient that you were "tired of hearing their complaints." On February 1, I again observed you yelling at a patient who forgot his checkbook. I sent you home for the remainder of the day without pay to consider if you still wanted your job. I told you to come back to work the following day with a written document of how you will correct the problem immediately. I once again suggested the services of the Employee Assistance Program and also registered you for a Conflict Management and Anger Management course at the local university that will begin on February 15. You are required to attend these courses as a condition of your continued employment at this practice.

I want to be sure you understand that I am seriously concerned about your performance. I expect you to be polite, understanding and helpful with every patient who walks into our office. If you are having problems at home that are interfering with your performance on the job, you must contact me to discuss options. If you are having family problems, you should continue to use our Employee Assistance Program. If you need some time off and want to use some of your accumulated vacation days, you should submit a request at least two days in advance.

A copy of this memo documenting your written warning will be placed in your personnel file. Unless improvement is immediate and sustained, you will be subject to further disciplinary action, up to and including termination.

I have received a copy of this memo and understand the context:

____

Joe Smith/Date

Documentation as Constructive Feedback

Ideally, feedback should be provided immediately and it's not always possible to do so. When feedback must be delayed, documentation provides managers and supervisors with the necessary reminders of what and when a specific incident occurred. Good feedback, based on strong documentation, helps employees to improve their behavior before it becomes a major problem. If poor performance becomes an ongoing challenge, documentation is necessary for a manager, supervisor, or human resource professional to defend any adverse actions taken.

Sometimes, employees having ongoing performance issues may need to be placed on a performance support plan. It provides a history of discussions and anticipated solutions and serves as a written log for managers or supervisors and employees. An example of a performance support form is provided in Figure 8-3. Performance support forms should be placed in the employee's personnel file.

Figure 8-3
EMPLOYEE PERFORMANCE SUPPORT PLAN

Name________________________ Job Title ____________________

To be completed by the manager:
Employee's performance has been unsatisfactory for the following reasons:

To be completed by BOTH manager and employee:
We have agreed upon the following steps that are necessary to correct these problem(s):

It is agreed that improvement in these areas must be **immediate and sustained**. We have also agreed that we will review this program on a weekly basis to discuss progress that has been made and any further action that may be necessary to complete the corrective action fully.

Employee Signature* ____________________ Date __________
Manager Signature* ____________________ Date __________
Human Resources ____________________ Date __________

* Signatures of employee and manager acknowledge that this situation has been discussed and that both parties agree to the plan of corrective action and that improvement must be immediate and sustained. The employee understands that failure to abide by this support plan satisfactorily will result in termination.

FOLLOW-UP REMARKS:

Employee Signature* ____________________ Date __________
Manager Signature* ____________________ Date __________

FOLLOW-UP REMARKS:

Employee Signature* ____________________ Date __________
Manager Signature* ____________________ Date __________

Source: Powers, Tara, Powers Training and Developmental Resources 2001

Documentation is important to ensure that employees are evaluated consistently and that all performance issues are managed fairly to protect both employees and the practice. Also remember that compliments and accomplishments should also be noted and maintained in personnel files.

Training Areas for Supervisors and Other Key People

- Diversity
- Retention
- Performance Management Process
- Coaching and Mentoring
- Recognition and Rewards

Training Supervisors and Other Key People

The Role of Managers and Supervisors in Retention and Effective Performance Management Systems

Managers and supervisors often underrate their roles in making performance management systems effective. Throughout this book, best practices and guidelines of implementing and managing the performance management process have been identified and explained in detail. Much of the performance interaction that takes place in your group practice will be between management and employees.

The role of managers and supervisors is so important; it actually goes beyond performance management. Managers have the major role in retaining talent in your organization. A recent report by the Conference Board of Canada in 2000 revealed that managers and supervisors are the major reason why employees leave.[8] Research conducted by Integral Training Systems, who specialize in retention strategies and management training, indicates that managers play a significant role in influencing employee commitment to the organization.

Managers influence employee productivity, the climate that encourages employees to commit and meet their goals, and whether employees receive meaningful feedback on their performance and behavior.[9] It's critical that training be provided to all managers, supervisors and other key people who have direct responsibility for measuring and managing employee performance.

Training Areas for Supervisors and Other Key People

For your performance management system to be successfully integrated, training should be provided in the following areas:

- Diversity—To provide awareness, understanding and management of accepting differences in the workplace, including age, gender, sexual orientation, education and religion.
- Retention—To learn their role in motivating and retaining employees.
- Performance Management Process—To understand the components of the system and how they interrelate. To have guidelines and practice in setting goals with employees, how to measure performance and provide effective performance reviews.
- Coaching and Mentoring—To learn the elements of an effective coach, become a better listener and provide constructive feedback and modeling.
- Recognition and Rewards—To learn guidelines for giving recognition and how to reward top performance in individuals and teams.

Each component of the performance management system requires managers and supervisors to perform their own roles effectively. Successful integration can't happen without them.

Two Phases of Evaluation

Phase I: Development and Implementation Evaluation

Phase II: Meeting System Objectives Evaluation

Evaluating and Revising Performance Systems

How will you know if your performance management system is meeting the needs of the group practice, managers and supervisors and your employees? The best way to improve a system is to evaluate it. Most organizations evaluate their systems on an annual basis; however, it is recommended that the first evaluation take place within the first six months of implementation.

The Two Phases of Evaluation

Other organizations that have conducted evaluations on their performance management system successfully recommend that an evaluation be done in two phases: first, evaluate the development and implementation of the system, and second, evaluate whether the objectives of the system have been met.

Start by creating an evaluation plan. Your plan should outline the objectives of the evaluation, the methods to be used, and the expected outcomes of the evaluation process. By outlining your plan with specific expected outcomes, evaluators can focus their efforts to effectively gather only the information they need. Examples of each part of the evaluation plan follow.

Sample objectives of the evaluation may include:

- To assess the implementation of the system to see if it provides the group practice with a results-focused employee evaluation system using relevant and measurable criteria linked to the goals of the practice;
- To assess how well the group practice is integrating the performance management system into other management initiatives; and
- To determine if managers, supervisors and employees see the performance management system as a means to provide communication about job performance and to recognize and reward, as well as evaluate, employee accomplishments.

Sample Evaluation Methods

Surveys—Distributed in manual form or electronically via e-mail to a representative sampling of managers, supervisors, human resource specialists and employees from different work areas.

On-site visits—Meet with various managers, supervisors, human resource specialists and employees from different work areas to:

- Review employee performance plans to determine if the plans are results-focused and link to practice objectives;
- Conduct focus groups or an individual interview to determine how well the performance management system is operating and whether it is achieving the desired outcomes.

Sample Desired Outcomes

- Employees, managers and supervisors understand the performance management process and the practice's system.

- Individual performance plans link with the practice's goals and objectives.
- Performance measures reflect and accurately review core factors important to the group practice's success.
- Feedback from managers and supervisors, employees, top management and/or other key people in the group practice indicate that the performance management system is easy to work with.
- Performance goals and objectives are being met.
- Employees feel they are being measured fairly.
- Managers and supervisors recognize and reward top performance.
- Employee satisfaction, attitude and morale are high.
- Managers and supervisors provide two-way communication and feedback on the effectiveness of the performance management system.
- Patients indicate satisfaction with their care and report that the group practice is meeting their needs.

A sample evaluation plan is provided in Figure 8-4.

Figure 8-4
Sample Performance Management System Evaluation Plan

Development and Implementation Questions for Employees:

- ❑ Were you involved in setting individual performance goals with your manager/supervisor?
- ❑ Did you and your manager/supervisor discuss your performance expectations and outcomes (results) to be achieved?
- ❑ Do you understand how your performance expectations support the group practice's goals?
- ❑ To what extent did the system affect the amount and quality of communication between you and your manager/supervisor?

Meeting Objectives of the System Questions for Employees:

- ❑ Did your manager/supervisor provide ongoing communication and feedback on your performance?
- ❑ Did your manager/supervisor provide constructive suggestions to improve your performance?
- ❑ Is your performance appraisal a fair reflection of your performance?
- ❑ Do you receive the training needed to perform your job effectively?
- ❑ Do you believe the performance management system allows employees to be recognized and rewarded for their performance?
- ❑ Has there been an improvement in your performance since the system was implemented?

Development and Implementation Questions for Managers/Supervisors:

- ❑ Are you confident in implementing each component of the Performance Management System, including aligning individual performance goals with the practice's, measuring employee performance, conducting performance reviews, providing coaching and feedback, and recognizing and rewarding performance?
- ❑ Are you confident in explaining how the performance expectations of your direct reports support the group practice's goals?
- ❑ Was each employee involved in setting his or her individual performance goals?
- ❑ Did you discuss performance expectations and outcomes (results) to be achieved with each employee?
- ❑ To what extent did the system affect the amount and quality of communication between you and your employees?

Meeting Objectives of the System Questions for Managers and Supervisors:

- ❑ Did you provide ongoing communication and feedback for each employee on his or her performance?
- ❑ Do you provide constructive suggestions to improve each employee's performance?
- ❑ Do you feel that performance appraisals provide a fair reflection of your employees' performance?
- ❑ Do you receive the training needed to develop and implement the system effectively?
- ❑ Do you believe the performance management system allows employees to be recognized and rewarded for their performance?
- ❑ Has there been an improvement in employee and/or unit performance since the system was implemented? [10]

Assessing the value and effectiveness of your performance management system is necessary for determining how to improve it. Planning for ongoing evaluation will allow your practice to revise it as needed. If you used initial surveys for customer satisfaction or other measures, they may also be used to compare levels between the old and new processes.

Chapter 6 in MGMA's book *Medical Practice Performance Management: How to Evaluate Employees,* offers additional tips on evaluating your performance management system.

Benefits to Using Online Systems

- Streamlines processes
- Provides assistance to evaluators
- Reduces time

Disadvantages to Using Online Systems

- Lack of technical expertise
- "Cookie-cutter" narratives
- Employee concerns

Using Online Performance Management Systems

Organizations use online performance management tools or entire systems for different reasons. For some, limited personnel resources and time allow them to do more with less. For others, it's an effort to streamline the process of performance management.

Benefits to Using Online Performance Management Systems

Many organizations use automated performance system applications to alleviate the tedious paper trail that a manual process involves. There are three primary advantages for using software applications for support performance management systems:

- They streamline the performance management process by compiling information, and providing records that can be e-mailed, making information accessible to other key people, and keeping documentation in one place;
- They provide assistance by suggesting sample sentences to reflect the rating assigned in performance appraisals and make word-processing editors available to personalize individual appraisals; and
- They reduce the amount of time it takes to do an appraisal by offering step-by-step instructions to help managers and supervisors write the performance plan, keep notes on a specific employee's performance, and finally rate the employee prior to his or her review.

Disadvantages to Using Online Performance Management Systems

- Users (managers, supervisors and employees) lack of technical expertise or have computer "phobia";
- Not all performance raters (co-workers, managers or supervisors) have access to computers or the Internet to use online applications;
- Employees receive "cookie-cutter" narratives of their performance because managers and supervisors don't personalize the appraisal; and
- Employees have concerns about security and privacy.[11]

Types of Online Evaluations

There are several different types of online performance management applications available in the market. Some organizations prefer to conduct a 360-degree assessment of employee performance. This type of assessment allows employees to receive feedback from their co-workers, managers and supervisors, and patients on how well they are meeting performance expectations. Core competencies of managers, supervisors and employees can be rated anonymously using this assessment tool. In all cases, it's important that group practices use tools that are statistically valid and reliable.

The Booth Company located in Boulder, CO, has developed 720-degree evaluations, called Task Cycle® Surveys, to reliably evaluate core competencies and behavior. According to Daniel Booth, president, "A 720-assessment provides a more accurate measure because the evaluation is actually done twice. Assessing employees at the beginning of a review period provides a baseline measure. Then, employees are reassessed six months or a year later to reflect performance and behavioral changes. It isn't fair to make assumptions when people have only been assessed once as many competencies may be newly developed."

The Booth Company has also developed an online leadership assessment that measures the effectiveness of managers and supervisors in the health care industry. A technical white paper, entitled, "Leadership in Health Services" is available for review from The Booth Company. Contact them at www.boothco.com.[12]

Total Performance Management Systems Available Online

Automated performance management systems provide a total solution for organizations of all sizes. These systems provide tools to create day-to-day feedback, help managers write meaningful performance reviews, and can even provide effective coaching strategies depending on the performance issue.

For example, one particular online package touts that it can do the following for your practice:

- Set, track and measure goals and objectives.
- Document day-to-day events and critical incidents to provide specific examples of performance for the review period.
- Provide valuable coaching ideas to help manage poor performers and challenge high achievers.
- Set reminders for upcoming reviews and documenting performance milestones.
- Link relevant documents from other programs to employees' records.
- Access past and present reviews for reference.
- Create customized worksheets for employee self-review and peer reviews.
- Shares reviews over the LAN to get feedback from other team members or managers.
- Create core competencies from a large database of descriptors.
- Compile forced-rating scores to determine an average rated score for each performance category.[13]

Examples of Online Performance Management Systems

- Performance Now Enterprise Edition – www.maus.com.
- 20/20 Insight® GOLD – www.2020insightgold.com.
- Panoramic Feedback – www.panoramicfeedback.com.
- Precision 360™ - www.teamsinc.com.
- Visual 360® - www.mindsolve.com.
- Corporate Pulse-Pulse Tools – www.vitalityalliance.com.
- Task Cycle® Surveys - www.boothco.com.

Information about each of these online applications can be accessed from their Web sites. You can also conduct a search on the Internet for reviews on these tools or ask other group practices which application they use and/or recommend.

Legal Cautions

Evaluating employee performance can trigger lawsuits. Managers and supervisors can reasonably expect that some evaluations will result in hurt feelings, defensive reactions and perhaps arguments. They may also result in lawsuits if employees feel they have been evaluated unfairly.

Lawsuits resulting from performance evaluations occur for various reasons. The following list cites several reasons an employee may sue an organization as a result of an evaluation.

When Performance Evaluations Trigger Lawsuits

- Untrue statements made in an evaluation are conveyed to a third party, such as co-workers or individuals in the community. The manager and organization may be sued for slander or libel.
- The employee feels that his or her manager intentionally inflicted emotional distress by the content or nature of the evaluation.
- The employee thinks that the evaluation resulted in his or her "wrongful" termination.
- The manager or supervisor used the evaluation to retaliate against the employee for something unrelated to the performance being reviewed.
- The manager or supervisor violated one of the anti-discrimination laws.
- An employee receives glowing performance evaluations and is never promoted or advanced in his or her career. The organization is thought to be biased toward employees of color, a certain age, gender, etc.
- An employee feels he or she is working under "hostile conditions" and is then wrongly discharged because of his or her complaints.
- The employee feels that his or her manager has been "building a case" against him or her.

Even though lawsuits may result in favor of the practice, the time, money, morale and public relations issues accompanying the litigation can be costly.[14]

The Truth about Evaluations and Lawsuits

- Performance evaluations can lead to lawsuits under state and federal anti-discrimination laws, as well as state tort theories like intentional infliction of emotional distress and defamation.
- Liability may result from both overly positive evaluations AND from overly negative ones. Saying too much and saying too little can have the same outcome.
- Managers and supervisors should be careful to ensure that any factual statements made during a performance evaluation are true. Information related to the evaluation should only be revealed to those who need to know.
- Performance evaluations backed with good documentation can be supported in a court of law. Managers and supervisors should make timely notes about behavior throughout an evaluation period.
- Most liability results from evidence of a pattern of evaluation that adversely affects employees in a protected class.[15]

How to Prevent Lawsuits from Performance Evaluations

Managers and supervisors, and all other evaluators of employee performance should be aware and keep abreast of employment laws as they relate to appraisals. A good source of information is *Tracking Hot HR Trends,* a MGMA 2001 publication. The chapter about tracking employment laws is a definite must-read to become more knowledgeable about current legislation as it relates to group practices.[16]

Use the following information as a quick reference guide on employment laws and how they relate to performance evaluations. Under each law or legal principle, there is a summary and a recommendation for protecting your practice in performance evaluation. Knowing the law and how managers and supervisors can prevent litigation against themselves and the group practice is the first step in prevention.

Employment Law Reference Guide

Employment at Will

Summary of the law/legal principle—The practice or employee may end the relationship at any time.

Recommendation for performance evaluations—Put "employment at will" clauses in job offers, employee handbooks and performance appraisals that employees sign prior to employment.

Implied Contract

Summary of the law/legal principle—The employment relationship has a non-explicit agreement that may impact some aspect of employment.

Recommendation for performance evaluations—Read and understand employment contracts that are non-standard in regard to evaluating performance.

Negligence

Summary of the law/legal principle—The practice breaches its duty to conduct performance appraisals timely and with due care.

Recommendation for performance evaluations—Keep employees advised if performance is poor so they can't contest a faulty evaluation process.

Defamation

Summary of the law/legal principle—The practice discloses untrue or unfavorable performance that damages an employee's reputation.

Recommendation for performance evaluations–Establish procedures to control or avoid providing false performance information (favorable or unfavorable).

Misrepresentation

Summary of the law/legal principle—The practice discloses untrue performance that causes risk or harm to others.

Recommendation for performance evaluations–Establish procedures to control or avoid providing false performance information (favorable or unfavorable).

Family and Medical Leave Act (FMLA)

Summary of the law/legal principle—The practice has an obligation to reinstate employees returning from leave to similar positions.

Recommendation for performance evaluations–Ensure that all managers and supervisors are knowledgeable about this law and any links to performance issues.

Disparate Treatment

Summary of the law/legal principle—The practice intentionally discriminates or has improper distinctions among employees based on protected status (e.g., race, gender, sexual orientation, age).

Recommendation for performance evaluations—Train managers and supervisors to avoid comments related to race, gender, religion, sexual orientation or age in verbal/written appraisals. Managers and supervisors should keep proper documentation on all performance issues.

Disparate (Adverse Impact)

Summary of the law/legal principle—The practice unintentionally discriminates from employment practices that appears neutral but affects those protected by discrimination law (e.g., race, gender, sexual orientation, age).

Recommendation for performance evaluations—Train managers and supervisors to avoid comments related to race, gender, religion, sexual orientation or age in verbal/written appraisals. Managers and supervisors should keep proper documentation on all performance issues.

Title VII of the Civil Rights Act of 1964 (Title VII)

Summary of the law/legal principle—The practice is outlawed from discrimination based on race, color, sex, religion or national origin.

Recommendation for performance evaluations—Train managers and supervisors to avoid comments related to race, gender, religion, sexual orientation or age in verbal/written appraisals. Managers and supervisors should keep proper documentation on all performance issues.

Equal Pay Act of 1963

Summary of the law/legal principle—The practice is prohibited from gender-based differences in pay for equal work, subject to limited exceptions.

Recommendation for performance evaluations—Train managers and supervisors to avoid comments related to gender in verbal/written appraisals. Managers and supervisors should keep proper documentation on all performance issues.

Civil Rights Act of 1991 (CRA 1991)

Summary of the law/legal principle—Jury trials, compensatory and punitive damages may result in discrimination cases. The burden of proof and other technical aspects may be altered in some cases.

Recommendation for performance evaluations—Train managers and supervisors to avoid comments related to race, gender, religion, sexual orientation or age in verbal/written appraisals. Managers and supervisors should keep proper documentation on all performance issues.

Age Discrimination in Employment Action (ADEA)

Summary of the law/legal principle—The practice is prohibited from employment discrimination based on those over the age of 40.

Recommendation for performance evaluations—Train managers and supervisors to avoid age-related comments in verbal/written appraisals; update performance criteria and training as technology changes to avoid claims that older workers are laid off for lack of newer skills.

Americans with Disabilities Act (ADA)

Summary of the law/legal principle—The practice is prohibited from employment discrimination based on disability.

Recommendation for performance evaluations—Review recommendations/appraisal results for evidence of discrimination; only essential functions should be evaluated; train managers and supervisors to identify reasonable accommodations, to focus on performance criteria and maintain sensitive or confidential information.[17]

Summary

Chapter 8 in MGMA's book *Medical Practice Performance Management: How to Evaluate Employees,* provides additional information on avoiding legal pitfalls in performance management.

Unfortunately, we live in a litigious society. Your practice should provide adequate training and knowledge about current state and federal laws and regulations to all managers and supervisors. Knowledge is prevention. Beyond training, random audits of performance appraisals are a good idea to check for compliance.

In this chapter, you reviewed six critical areas to evaluate your performance management system integration. Planning and implementing preventive measures in these areas will not only ensure its success; it will save you valuable time and minimize legal challenges.

References:

1. Dick Grote, "The Secrets of Performance Appraisal: Best Practices from the Masters," Zigon Performance Group, www.zigonperf.com.

2. Robert Bacal, "A Quick Guide to Employee Orientation—Help for Managers and HR," www.work911.com, 2000.

3. Oak Ridge National Laboratory, www.ornl.gov.

4. Robert Bacal, "A Quick Guide to Employee Orientation—Help for Managers and HR," www.work911.com, 2000.

5. *Disciplining Employees,* Business & Legal Reports, Inc. 1997.

6. Mary Cook, *The Complete Do-It-Yourself Human Resources Department,* Prentice-Hall, 2001.

7. Oak Ridge National Laboratory, www.ornl.gov.

8. Keepers, Inc., www.keepersinc.com.

9. Integral Training Systems, www.itsinc.net.

10. Dick Grote, "The Secrets of Performance Appraisal: Best Practices from the Masters," Zigon Performance Group, www.zigonperf.com.

11. "Department of Transportation Evaluates Its Performance Management System," Workforce Performance Newsletter, October 1998, www.opm.gov.

12. Daniel Booth, The Booth Company, www.boothco.com.

13. "Automating Performance Management," Workforce Performance Newsletter, February 1999, www.opm.gov.

14. MAUS Business Systems, www.maus.com.

15. Mary-Kathryn Zachary, "Performance Evaluations Trigger Many Lawsuits," Zigon Performance Group, August 2000, www.zigonperf.com.

16. Alys Novak and Courtney Price, T*racking Hot HR Trends: The Group Practice Personnel Policies Update,* MGMA, Englewood, CO, 2001.

17. Stanley B. Malos, J.D., "Current Legal Issues in Performance Appraisal," www.cob.sjsu.edu.

Tips for Successful Performance Management

Chapter 9

Implementing a successful performance system in any practice starts with the role of the supervisor. It is important to determine how supervisory skills impact the performance level of employees.

As a supervisor or manager, your leadership style can have a positive or negative influence on the success of your employees and the practice. The key question: Are you developing a sense of personal and professional satisfaction in the performance of your employees?

How you communicate with your employees also says a lot about your effectiveness as a leader. Do you have an open and honest relationship with your team?

Are you skillful in the art of persuasion and influence to build commitment in your employees?

Are you confident that you are communicating clear expectations to your employees and that goals of the practice will most likely be achieved?

In this chapter we will attempt to answer these important questions, give you new ideas to implement, and hopefully get you thinking about how you can be more successful in your leadership role in order to improve the performance of your employees. We will cover important areas such as:

- Effective leadership techniques;
- Assessment of leadership skills;
- "Walking the talk" as a leader;
- Gaining employee commitment;
- The importance of communication; and
- Managing employee expectations.
-

Leadership

Leadership is defined as *having the ability to influence others to act in a particular way.*[1] Leaders in any organization can come in all shapes and sizes, holding various positions in the organization. An individual does not necessarily have to supervise others to be considered a leader, rather he or she could emerge from within a team or group. On the other hand, in most organizations it is expected that a manager or supervisor exhibit leadership qualities. Since all leaders must have followers, one of the most important questions a manager can ask is "Would I follow myself?"

Basic Principles of Effective Leadership

1. No "One" Right Answer
2. Effective Decisions the First Time
3. Sensitivity to Others
4. Leadership Style for the Situation

The Role of Effective Leadership in Performance Management

In any practice, for a leader to impact change, create a motivated workforce, build effective teams, ensure excellent customer service, and increase productivity, employee performance must be managed appropriately.

As a leader, you have the opportunity to influence others to achieve goals, maximize performance, accept challenges, and be the best they can be. Since today's workplace is constantly changing, being a responsive and flexible leader is critical to successful performance management. To be effective, leaders need to adapt their styles to suit a broad range of individual and team performance situations especially with a multi-generational workforce. For more information on how to manage the performance of different generations at work, please review Chapter 1 on the increasingly diverse workforce.

According to Ken Blanchard, a leading organizational theorist, effective leadership is being able to adapt leadership behavior to the meet the performance needs of the individual or group.[2] Listed now are some pointers that can be used as guidelines for adapting effective leadership techniques for different situations:

- Realize there can be a *variety of solutions* for any given situation. However, some solutions will be more effective in reaching desired outcomes than others. For example, one employee may only need additional training to perform exceptionally where another employee may be in the wrong job based on his or her qualifications.

- Make an *effective decision* the first time or the performance problem or issue may grow larger and more difficult to handle. If you choose the right solution for the problem, you will be much more effective than if you just throw out a "quick fix" for the short term.

- *Be sensitive* to individual performance needs and tailor leadership styles accordingly. Some employees need more guidance then others. Some employees may need more of a personal touch so that they know you care. This could be as easy as stopping by their desk each morning to say "hello."

- According to Ken Blanchard a good leader uses *different leadership styles* in different situations.[2] Depending on individual/team performance needs, time constraints, and resources, a leader can act as:

    a. A *director* if the employee or team needs be told exactly what to do and how to do it. This is usually appropriate when the employee or team is a new hire or is new to the process or team. They need to be shown what to do and clear directions on how to do it right.

    b. A *coach* who can help an employee or team understand the plan and then coach them on action steps along the way. This type of style is used when an employee or team knows how to do the job but does not have the initiative or confidence to get the job done. The leader needs to act as coach and motivator helping to develop positive attitudes toward reaching goals.

c. A *supporter* who is available to help employees and teams make important decisions only if needed. Leaders should use this style when employees know how to get the job done. They are motivated to reach the goals but they may have some questions along the way. The leader's job is to be a supportive resource when needed.

d. A *delegator* who only has to say to an experienced and knowledgeable employee or team "go to it." This is the most desirable style for any leader. This style is used when the employee is highly skilled and highly motivated. The employee only needs is to be empowered to make decisions and will reach the goal on his or her own.

Do you have what it takes to be an effective leader? The following assessment will take a look at leadership skills that are necessary to be effective and help you determine areas where you could improve.

Assessment of Leadership Skills

Instructions: The following skills have been identified as skills for effective leadership. Use the scale to rate your skill level. Place your answer next to the question in the far left margin.

When completed with the assessment, choose three – four areas that you need to work on to become a more effective leader. Develop personal goals to improve these skills and identify resources that will help you accomplish your goals (i.e., additional training, partnering with a mentor, etc). Please see the resources included at the end of this chapter for additional information on leadership training courses.

RATING SCALE

Never
1
Rarely
2
Occasionally
3
Frequently
4
All the time
5

Leadership Traits[3]

1. I have a strong desire to complete tasks or reach goals and will put forth 110 percent effort to make sure they happen.
2. I have high standards and high expectations of myself and my employees.
3. I willingly take initiative on developing steps toward reaching goals or completing tasks.
4. I accept responsibility for a variety of tasks and have a strong desire to motivate others to complete their tasks.
5. Those who work with me view me as trustworthy and honest.
6. I am confident in my abilities and I am not afraid to convince others of goals and decisions that I feel are correct.
7. I understand my role and the role of my employees and have the knowledge and experience to solve problems and make good decisions.

People Skills

1. I listen to my employees and try to understand their feelings summarizing what was said and asking questions to clarify when needed.
2. I have respect for various opinions and views even if they are different from my own.
3. I provide feedback that is honest, helpful and understood.
4. I give recognition as often as I can by catching people doing something right.
5. I inspire others to believe in the organizational mission and develop a shared vision with those I work with.
6. I elicit information and ideas by asking open-ended questions.
7. I act as a mediator when necessary, helping employees or co-workers work out an agreement or a solution.
8. I develop a supportive environment by showing interest in the well being and success of my employees and co-workers.

Effectiveness Skills

1. I help employees stay on track toward the achievement of goals by following up, continually involving employees in decision making, and making certain to celebrate milestone accomplishments.
2. I clarify expectations or goals when needed.
3. I help employees set priorities and plan action steps toward reaching goals.
4. I initiate ideas, actions, solutions and procedures when needed.
5. I communicate ideas effectively making sure that everyone understands.
6. I influence people to develop action plans toward a successful solution.
7. I ask appropriate questions when information is not clear or understandable.
8. I analyze ideas, tasks or processes to determine if they will be effective in solving the problem.
9. I recognize roadblocks or obstacles to implementing a new idea.
10. I evaluate and measure progress toward reaching goals.
11. My actions and behavior serve as a role model to my employees.

Source: Powers, Tara. Powers Training & Developmental Resources, 2001.

How To "Walk the Talk" as a Leader

1. Build Trust.
2. Develop Open Communication Channels.
3. Empower Others.
4. Motivate Staff.
5. Measure Employee Satisfaction.
6. Partner With Employees.

How To "Walk the Talk" In Your Practice

To have a successful practice, you must implement and carry out effective leadership skills. To do this, effective leaders must take an active role in:

1. *Building trust* – Honesty and credibility are essential to leadership. If employees are going to follow you, they first want to assure themselves that you can be trusted. When employees have trust in you as a leader, they will believe in your decisions and actions because they are confident that you are doing what is best for them and the practice. You can build trust by taking an interest in your employees, meeting with them on a regular basis, and doing what you say you are going to do.

2. *Communicating openly* – Constantly developing improved ways of communicating with and listening to the staff. This can be done in a variety of ways including weekly staff meetings where employee have 10 minutes to discuss any issues, suggestion boxes, one-on-one meetings, etc.

3. *Empowering others* – Delegating tasks and handing over decision making to an employee or team that is motivated and committed to perform, is a critical piece in establishing value and ownership. However, it is important that employees and team members are confident and able to perform acceptably.

4. *Motivating staff* – Motivation is the key to gaining commitment toward achieving goals. However, it is important to note that each individual is influenced and motivated by different factors. A leader should take time to understand what really excites employees. It could be financial reward, recognition, opportunity for growth and development, or training that helps to create a motivated environment. (Please see Chapter 7 for more information on rewarding and recognizing employees.)

5. *Measuring levels of employee satisfaction* – Through discussions, employee self-evaluations, annual surveys, etc., leaders will have a better understanding of how employees feel and can partner with employees to implement

changes. Resources on-line to help your practice develop surveys can be found at:

- www.inquisite.com
- www.surveymonkey.com

6. *Partnering with employees* – Ideally, the whole relationship between leader and employee should be a partnership where together leaders and employees develop action steps that can be taken to make positive changes in the work environment. This can be done during performance appraisals, feedback discussions, or weekly staff meetings where leaders give employees the chance to articulate their own ideas and plans on how to reach goals, solve problems and improve processes in the workplace.

Commitment

Employees committed to the strategic goals and success of the practice will ensure your survival as an organization. Clear, positive images of the future of the practice and how it will continue to meet employee's needs must be created. Employees should understand the strategic goals of the practice for the next two to five years. This creates a vision in the employee's mind that the organization plans on being around for a while and that the employee's skills may be needed for years to come.

Employees are also interested in how the practice is planning on keeping up with changes in the marketplace. For example, does the Human Resources department pay attention to cost-of-living adjustments, market salaries for similar employee jobs? Are the practice's benefits in-line with other top practices in the country? What type of recognition and reward programs are being offered at other group practices?

Happy, engaged, committed employees will impact your bottom line and increase customer loyalty. Having a practice where employees are valued and respected, pay is equitable and fair, recognition is given for hard work, and employees feel part of a team, will instill commitment and will influence retention, customer satisfaction and the overall success of the practice.

"All For One and One For All"

It can be a difficult task getting all of your employees committed to working together and achieving the goals of the practice. However, employees will be more willing to work harder and support one another in the achievement of organization-wide goals if they have the following:

- ✓ A positive attitude about the practice they work for;
- ✓ A perceived notion that their contributions are valued and recognized;
- ✓ A feeling that the practice genuinely cares about them;
- ✓ A sense of team camaraderie and support; and
- ✓ A voice when instituting change.

To develop a organization where all employees are committed to a common goal and will work together toward achieving that goal, an organization should follow these guidelines:

- Design a recognition and reward program that motivates your team to work together to be successful.
- Inspire and challenge your team to do great work by setting an example and always doing your best at whatever you do.
- Involve the team in decision making whether it be about performance goals and expectations, how to be more effective or productive, or a reward program for doing a good job.
- Provide appropriate rewards to teams who achieve objectives.

By encouraging a sense of belonging, team members will be motivated to take on team goals, particularly when the message of commitment is delivered in a way that emphasizes individual and team benefits.

Factors That Influence Employee Commitment

1. Communication
2. Diversity
3. Job Satisfaction
4. Empowerment
5. Managerial Effectiveness
6. Work-Life Balance
7. Career Advancement

Enrolling Others for Commitment

Research shows that employers can impact the commitment level of their employees by creating a work environment that shows through action that the employee is valued. Pay is only one important part. There are many factors other than compensation that can influence employee commitment. In research conducted by WFD, Inc., the nation's leading HR consulting and research firm specializing in workplace improvement, many factors other than money were found to drive workforce commitment.[4]

Analyze the following factors to determine if your practice has set up an environment that encourages commitment:

- *Communication* – Is vertical and horizontal communication in your practice effective and acceptable to employees? Do employees willingly go to their managers with questions about something they don't understand? Are employees encouraged to discuss new ideas to improving processes and procedures? Are employees informed on how the practice is doing financially?

  - Employees should feel like they understand where the practice is heading and should be prepared for any upcoming changes to policies or procedures.

- *Diversity and Inclusion* – Do all employees in your practice feel they are treated fairly and equitably by the practice and by co-workers? Are there complaints or rumors of harassment or discrimination? Are some employees singled out because they are "different"?

  - Recognize individual differences – understand that no two employees are the same and each will have different needs. Learning to recognize those needs will ensure that each employee is treated fairly.

  - Check for equity – Individual rewards and recognition should be perceived as fair based on the effort that is presented regardless of race or gender. Proper rewards should be established based on what is important and valued by employees. Looking at your compensation structure on a regular basis, the job responsibilities of each employee, and determining if employees are being paid fairly for their work is an important part of managing diversity and meeting the requirements for equal employment opportunity.

- *Job satisfaction* – Are employees challenged by their job? Are learning opportunities available? Do employees have the resources to be effective?

  - Fair Pay – Employees should be paid fairly and equitably for the job they perform. This could include salary, merit increases, benefits and bonuses. The practice should stay abreast of what the market is paying for similar jobs. Any practice can subscribe to national, regional or industry surveys. Resources can be found at:

    - http://www.pohly.com/salary.html (health care salary and compensation survey information)
    - http://jobstar.org/tools/salary/salhelth.htm (includes nursing, physician, laboratory, patient care and other healthcare surveys)
    - http://www.hfma.org/career/salary.htm

  - Match employee to job – Ensure that employee preferences and capabilities are a good fit for the position.

    Example: Some employees do best working alone while others in a team environment. Some employees enjoy working with little supervision; others need direction and support to succeed. To determine this information, working with instrumental learning tools such as the Myers-Briggs Personality Type Indicator (MBTI) or the DISC Behavioral Profile may provide important information that will help the determine the type of environment an employee would excel in. These learning tools can be found online or through contacting any local training organization in your area.

  - Set challenging goals – Employees will be motivated to achieve goals when they are clearly communicated, measurable and the employee has helped to establish them. Achieving a goal gives the employee a sense of personal satisfaction and accomplishment.

- *Empowerment* – Do employees feel empowered to make decisions on how they perform their jobs?
    - Encourage participation – If employees are involved in making decisions that will affect their work, they are more willing to take ownership for the outcome of those decisions. Ownership can impact commitment and motivation.

- *Managerial Effectiveness* – Does the manager of the practice have the necessary leadership and people skills to be effective? Have you asked employees how they feel through the use of a survey or even a confidential 360 degree performance review of the manager? A 360 degree performance review is a tool used to assess the all-around effectiveness of an employee or manager. It allows for evaluation by a select group of the employee's peers, co-workers, subordinates, managers, and customers. This type of review paints a clear picture of the employee overall performance. Resources for 360 degree performance reviews can be found online or through any local training organization. "Off the shelf" software for this type of evaluation can also be found in any computer software store.

- *Work-Life Balance* – Is the practice flexible when dealing with personal and family obligations of employees?

    - Flexible work schedules may be something to consider when trying to meet employee needs.

- *Career Advancement* – Do employees feel that opportunities for advancement and growth exist in the practice?

Strategies for improving commitment in your practice could include an employee satisfaction survey that addresses the areas just discussed. Surveys can be custom-made to ask the questions that you need answers to and is a good measurement tool to help you decide where to focus efforts. Additional resources can be found at:

http://www.custominsight.com/employee-satisfaction-surveys.html
http://www.busreslab.com/evalue2.htm
http://www.employeesurveys.com/

Remember: If employees are committed, the practice will have a greater chance of reaching its goals, achieving optimal success, and creating a great place to work!

Communication

We live in a technological era where almost all communication can be done from a distance without any face-to-face contact. However, it should not be surprising that employees still rank face-to-face communication as the most effective and preferred communication technique to close gaps between managers and employees.[5]

What Do Employees Need to Know?

In survey after survey on communication in the workplace, employees have clearly stated that they need certain types of information to be communicated.[6] Included among the top topics are:

- ✓ Information required to do their job correctly;
- ✓ Knowledge of where their job fits into the overall "big picture";
- ✓ Information about the future direction of the organization
- ✓ Reasons for change in the work environment ; and
- ✓ Changes that will affect their performance and the opportunity for input.

Although most organizations realize that communication can be critical to success, employee satisfaction surveys many times have shown that communication is not always being handled at the level desired by employees. As a manager, it is important to understand your role in practicing effective organizational communication with employees.

Poor communication is a frequent cause of problems and resentment in the workplace. It is critical to verify that the message received is clearly the same as the message sent. This can be accomplished through using examples, citing similar situations, and assessing employee reactions to the message. Are employees excited about the information they have received or are employees reacting with stunned looks and silence? Another important point to remember is that communication must be appropriate to the audience. People must be given as much information as they need to ensure understanding. Too much information can lead to confusion, a feeling of being overwhelmed or even fear. Sometimes deciding on how much information to give to employees can be difficult to balance.

Encourage Communication Through:

1. Open-Ended Questions
2. Active Listening
3. Providing Feedback

The Role of Communication in Performance Management Systems

Communication is considered a key skill when managing the performance of your employees. Messages regarding performance expectations, goals and preferred behaviors must be communicated clearly and simply.

An essential part of communication in any performance management system is to gain the commitment of the employee or team in accomplishing their goals or expectations. This can be accomplished by using:

- *Open-ended questions* in any performance discussion between a supervisor and employee. Employees cannot answer open-ended questions with a simple yes or no but have to engage in communication with their manager. Examples of these questions include: "What obstacles do you feel might get in the way of achieving this goal?" "How do you think we could overcome these obstacles?" "What can we do together to resolve this problem?" Such questions can encourage employee ownership and a feeling of being valued.
- *Active listening skills* where you focus intently on what the employee is saying, empathize with the speaker by imagining being in his or her place, refrain from using judgment even when in disagreement, and ensure that you received and understood the intended meaning of the communication by asking questions that clarify the information.
- *Positive and corrective feedback* used to let employees know how they are doing. This is critical to the achievement of overall organizational goals, motivating employees and addressing performance problems early on. (For more information on using feedback appropriately, refer to Chapter 5, How To Enhance Employee Performance Through Feedback.)

Types of Communication

- Oral
- Written
- Electronic
- Nonverbal

How To Communicate Performance Results

There are many ways to communicate performance results to individuals or a team. Communicating results is an important step in helping employees understand how they are performing against expectations. As the supervisor or manager, you will have to decide on a case-by-case basis which type of communication will work best in any given situation. Some examples of ways to communicate feedback are listed now.

Oral Communication - This type of communication is the most personal and can have the greatest impact. Therefore, oral communication should be done as frequently and often as possible. Oral communication can build trust and create a supportive and open environment. It can take place face-to-face, in departmental staff meetings, or over the telephone.

Written Communication - Use this type of communication if the message is formal, detailed or important for future reference. Examples of written communication could include company newsletters, employee publications, policies or procedures, performance reviews, or anything that should have proper documentation. Written communication is also important when documenting employee performance or behaviors to be used to measure performance throughout the year. (For more information on the importance of documentation for performance management purposes, please see Chapter 8, Using Proper Documentation Techniques.)

Electronic Communication - Today you can use a variety of electronic media to communicate with your employees including e-mail, voicemail, paging, Internet, intranet and more. Using electronic communication is a great way to reach a number of people in a short period of time. Although it's quick and easy to use, it may not be the best communication tool for establishing appropriate relationships with your employees. However, it can be a great tool if a supervisor needed to outline action steps to an employee for an important project, or to follow up with an employee once goals have been established to see how he or she is doing.

Nonverbal Messages - Body language or voice tones can speak volumes and can be more meaningful than any other type of communication. They can communicate emotions or temperaments and can have a significant impact on employee performance. Be aware of the nonverbal messages that you may be sending. The nonverbal messages you send through body language can have a significant impact on employee satisfaction and can affect performance. Table 9.1 shows some typical body language and the messages that it can convey.

Figure 9.1
Typical Body Language

Attitude
Center
Facial Expression
Gestures
Posture

Disapproval or disagreement
Closed
Frown
Holding finger by nose;
shaking head; fists are hidden; crossed arms
Crossed legs, make look more tense than normal

Ready to make a decision
Open
Expectant
Tugging or touching clothes; looks ready to get up, hands placed on hips
Sitting on edge of chair, as though waiting to leave

Wants to terminate the conversation
Turned away; feet or body turned towards the exit
Seems mildly interested
Wringing or wiping hands; looking at watch or other jewelry
Disengaged or looking away from you

Bored
Closed
Blank look
Foot tapping or playing with a pen
Holding head with hands

Doesn't understand
Concave
Puzzling
Foot tapping or a blank look
Slumped over

Confident
Open
Excited
Strong eye contact; feet placed on desk; chin forward
Sitting erectly, arms behind head

Suspicious
Turned away; feet or body turned towards the exit
Scowl or eyes narrowed
Eyes squinting, arms crossed, wringing hands
Leaning back or staring directly
Wants to speak
Leaning toward sender
Nods in agreement
Touching other person
Leaning forward or toward sender

Nervous
Turned away
Tense or uptight
Playing with coins in pocket, clearing throat; covering mouth with hand; rubbing neck; running fingers through hair
Crossed arms or legs

Source: Hight, Cathi, HighTec Consulting Inc., 2001.

Managing Expectations

1. Identify.
2. Define Responsibility.
3. Agree.
4. Communicate.
5. Perform.
6. Measure .

Managing Expectations

Managing employee expectations is one of the most important steps in the performance management process. Expectations not only help new employees understand what is expected of them but also establish an objective basis for communicating with employees about performance. Expectations help employees differentiate between acceptable and unacceptable results and can increase job satisfaction when employees know they are performing well. Furthermore, expectations can encourage an open and trusting relationship between a manager and employee.
Listed now are some general guidelines to follow when managing employee expectations. Using these guidelines will help you achieve optimal results from your employees and enable you to meet the objectives of the practice:[7]

Identify: The first step in managing expectations is to identify what level of performance is expected in each particular job role. The manager should have the experience and knowledge to identify these expectations clearly through the personal experience of performing the job, by sitting side by side with the employee and observing how the job is done, or by being involved in training to ensure job knowledge.

Define Responsibility: Collaborate with employees on the development of individual performance expectations in performance planning meetings. Working together, develop expectations that move the employee's efforts in the direction of achieving specific results or goals that will benefit the practice. As we have discussed in Chapter 5, Implementing a Performance Management System, expectations should support organizational growth as well as the employee's professional growth.

Reach Agreement: To ensure success, employee and supervisor need to agree on the expectations that have been developed. It is possible that throughout the year, expectations may change if the job changes, the practice procedures change or there is a change in industry or governmental regulations. Any change in expectations need to be agreed upon by both manager and employee.

Communicate: At anytime the manager and employee can hold a meeting to revisit performance expectations and ensure that employees are achieving the identified results. This meeting might be initiated by the supervisor if the supervisor feels the employee is starting to head off track. (Please refer to Chapter 4, Coaching For Performance for additional information on how to use coaching to improve performance.) A meeting may also be initiated by the employee if the employee needs further clarification on goals or needs some additional information from the supervisor.

Either way, by communicating openly with employees on an ongoing basis about how they are doing in meeting expectations, employees are more likely to be successful in achieving the desired outcome when they understand exactly what they need to do and how they need to get there.

Perform: Once employees understand and agree with the expectations that have been jointly developed with supervisor, they can go for it! At this point, the job of the supervisor or manager is to be available for support, encouragement or to act as a coach if needed. Management will periodically report to employees on their progress using communication techniques outlined earlier in this chapter. They will work with employees on any developmental or training needs, and they will measure employee's performance against the established expectations to assess how the employee has performed throughout the year.

Communicating Expectations

Managers must clearly communicate the skills, behaviors and performance levels that employees are expected to demonstrate. When you communicate clear, understandable and agreeable expectations to your employees, you are creating an environment where employees can succeed. It is only in this type of environment where the organization will reach its goals, employee morale will be high, and hard work will be noticed and recognized.

Suggestion

Have your staff complete this questionnaire on you.

Communicating Expectations

This management questionnaire can be used as a tool to determine if you are properly communicating expectations to your employees. By honestly answering each question, you will understand if you doing a good job of establishing expectations with employees in your practice.

1. As a manager, I clearly communicate performance expectations to employees?
2. I work together with my employees to agree on performance expectations?
3. I set expectations and goals that challenge employees?
4. I work to gain commitment from employees when setting expectations?
5. My employees understand how their performance expectations support organizational objectives?
6. I measure performance results on a continual basis and communicate results to employees?
7. I help employees determine priorities?
8. I help employees implement action steps when needed to achieve expectations or goals?

If you have answered YES to most of these questions, you are effectively setting expectations with employees.

If some of your answers were NO, you may want to examine your procedures on setting expectations with employees. Employees should have clearly defined goals and expectations that tie in to the overall goals and objectives of the practice. Clear goals and expectations provide motivation for employees because they understand how they "fit" in the bigger picture and clearly see how they add value.

Source: Powers, Tara, Powers Training & Developmental Resources, 2001.

Measuring Expectations

Performance expectations are the basis for evaluating employee performance. Measuring expectations can help to identify areas that need development, or small, incremental changes that provide opportunities to reward improvements.[8]

To measure expectations a manager must continually gather performance data that is available and analyze the gap between what is expected and what actually happened. Performance data can be gathered through:

- Direct observation of performance.
  - Timing: This should be done on a daily basis
- Tangible work results such as client paperwork, data entry, etc.
  - Timing: This should be done at least monthly.
- Organizational records such as attendance records, insurance claim records, patient records.
  - Timing: This should be done on a quarterly basis, or if the need arises because an employee is not meeting expectations.
- Kudos, complaints or any other feedback received from co-workers, patients, suppliers or other supervisors.
  - Timing: Anytime they are given.

Performance data can be expressed in terms of quantity, quality, time, cost, effect, manner of performance, or method of performing.

Ways to measure performance expectations are:

- **Quantity:** describes how much work must be completed within a specified time; e.g., makes 10 appointments each day.

- **Quality**: specifies how well the work must be done. Can describe accuracy, precision, appearance or effectiveness; e.g., 90 percent of insurance claims are accepted without revision.

- **Timeliness:** answers the questions when is it needed by, how soon or within what period; e.g., all new patient paperwork completed within 24 hours.

- **Cost:** used when you can assess performance in terms of money saved, processing errors reduced, number of duplicate claims reduced, etc.

- **Results of effort:** addresses the results to be obtained; e.g., establish back-up plans so that client appointments are on-time 80 percent of the time.

- **Approach to performance:** describes circumstances where an individual's approach or behavior has an effect on performance; e.g., assists clients with any questions or concerns in a helpful and pleasant manner.

- **Method or policy for performing assignments:** describes requirements for any official policy or procedures for accomplishing the work; e.g., insurance forms are completed in accordance with established office procedures.

Summary

Conclusion

Successfully managing the performance of your employees requires you to look at your management skills as a leader, communicator, influencer and partner. By making a commitment to improving at least two skills discussed in this chapter, you will establish better relationships with your employees and create a culture in your practice that supports success.

References:

1. Stephen P. Robbins and David A. De Cenzo, *Supervision Today!* , Prentice-Hall, Inc, 2001.
2. On-line: http://www.triangle.org/leadership/sitlead.html
3. Stephen P. Robbins and David A. De Cenzo, *Supervision Today!* , Prentice-Hall, Inc, 2001.
4. On-line: http://www.wfd.com/press/pressreleases/9809wfdresearch.htm
5. On-line: http://www.iabc.com/events/f2f/why.htm
6. On-line: http://hrweb.berkeley.edu/guide/performance.htm
7. On-line: http://www.wfd.com/press/pressreleases/9809wfdresearch.htm
8. On-line: http://hrweb.berkeley.edu/guide/performance.htm

Additional Resources:

R. Bhasin, “Communicating With Employees” *Pulp and Paper Magazine* (November, 1999).

The Manager’s Bookshelf: A Mosaic of Contemporary Views. Jon Pierce & John Newstrom, HarperCollins College Publishers, 1996.

Patrick D. Lynch, Rober Eisenberger and Stephen Armeli, Perceived Organizational support: Inferior Versus Superior Performance by Wary Employees, Journal of Applied Psychology 1999

http://www.jobchannel.tv/recruiters/leadership.asp

http://www.nokia.com/insight/social/employee_commitment.html

Leadership Training Courses:

www.lessonsinleadership.com
http://www.padgettthompson.com/
http://www.amanet.org/index.htm
www.skillpath.com

Summing Up

"Hospitals, clinics, and other health care facilities across the United States are experiencing a common consequence of the pressure to contain costs. Fewer personnel are being used to accomplish a given work load, or the current staff is being asked to do more. The result is an increased, frequently more complex workload involving greater numbers of patients and carried out by fewer employees.

"In today's work environment, more than ever, supervisors need accurate measures of employee performance to gauge whether or not subordinates are performing their jobs at optimal levels of quality and quantity."'

—Anderson and Pulich[1]

Good performance management systems don't happen by accident. Consideration and planning are needed and critical elements must be in place to measure employee performance effectively. In this book, you explored the latest strategies and best practices in implementing and managing a performance management system and its processes.

Successful models start with aligning organizational goals to individual performance plans. Understanding and embracing performance management is a collaborative effort between the leadership, management and employees.

The need for developing and implementing a strong performance contract that provides winning outcomes throughout the organization has never been greater as medical practices face formidable challenges in the new century.

An effective performance management system makes it easier for managers and supervisors to discuss expectations and results with their direct reports. Employees clearly know what's expected from them and understand their impact on the organization's goals and outcomes. The real win for employees is being recognized and rewarded for top performance. This is the critical link between employees who work with the group practice to meet its goals, and feel valued and compensated fairly.

Performance management starts with clearly defined goals and expectations and creates results such as improved communication, team building, strategic partnerships, high morale and retention, and most of all, quality patient care.

In this manual, you have learned that a performance management system is more than appraisals and evaluations. It's an integrated way to share goals, measure what's important for success, provide ongoing and meaningful dialogue, and celebrate results. Your practice benefits in every area of its operations, your staff likes what they do, and your patients' expectations are exceeded. What better reasons do you need to invest the time and resources to have the best performance management system working for your medical practice?

References

1. Peggy Anderson and Marcia Pulich, "Making Performance Appraisals Work More Effectively," Health Care Advisor, 6/01/98, www.zigonperf.com.